WELL+GOOD

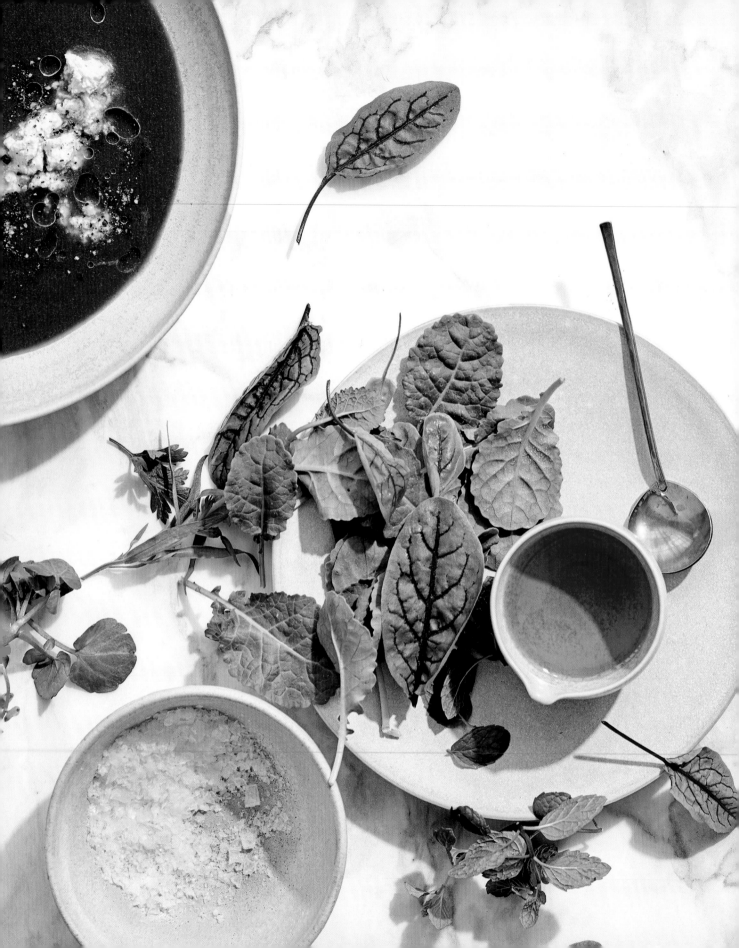

ALEXIA BRUE + MELISSE GELULA

WELL + GOOD

100 Healthy Recipes + Expert Advice for Better Living

Photography by

JOHNNY MILLER

CLARKSON POTTER/PUBLISHERS

NEW YORK

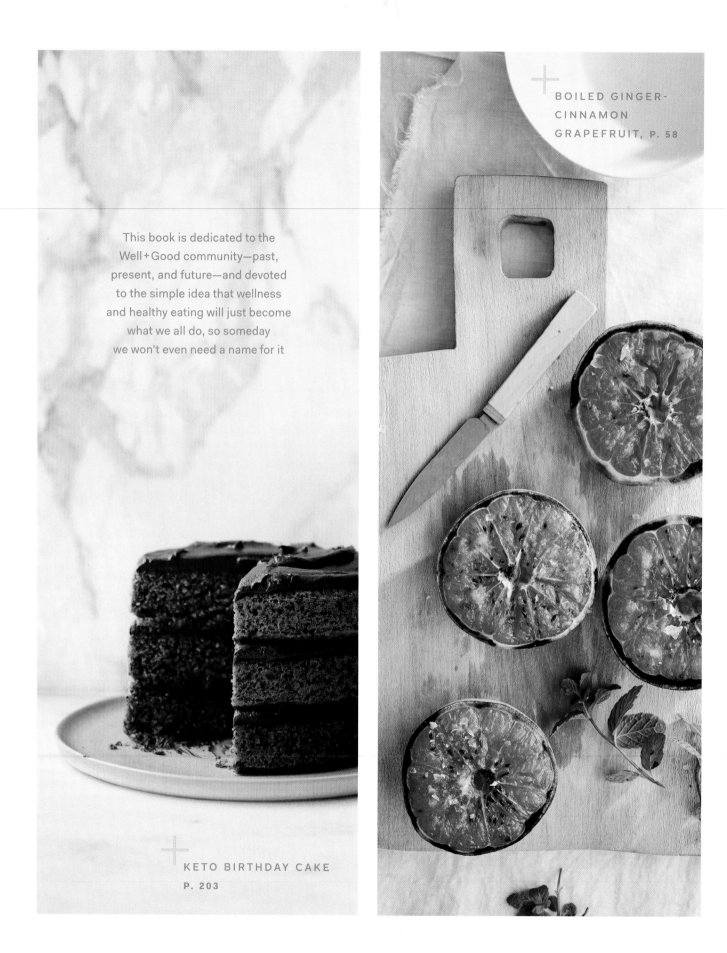

This book is dedicated to the
Well+Good community—past,
present, and future—and devoted
to the simple idea that wellness
and healthy eating will just become
what we all do, so someday
we won't even need a name for it

BOILED GINGER-
CINNAMON
GRAPEFRUIT, P. 58

KETO BIRTHDAY CAKE
P. 203

CONTENTS

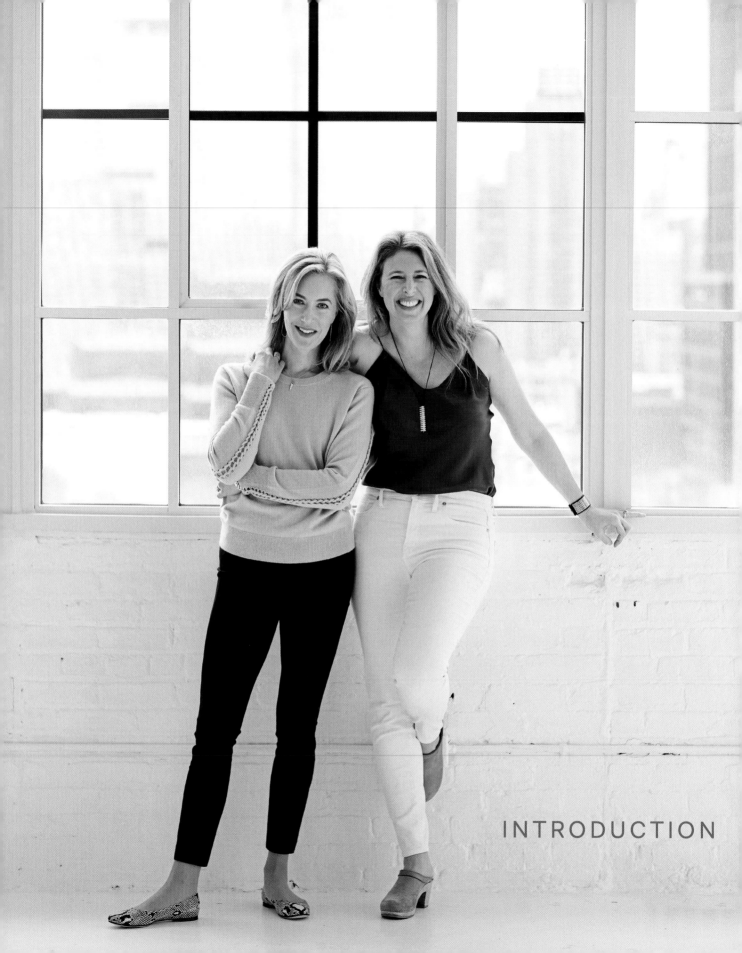

INTRODUCTION

Well+Good launched in the summer of 2009. We had a grand total of two staffers—Alexia and Melisse—and relied on the free Wi-Fi at New York City's Jivamukti Yoga Café (many, many green smoothies and grain bowls were consumed as thanks). We were two thirty-something journalists, who'd left our careers in magazines to start a website devoted to the burgeoning wellness scene, which, at the time, no other company was covering in a detailed or dedicated way.

For context: During this time, the healthy food scene was just beginning to pop. Whole Foods was opening more locations, and an intense interest in where our ingredients came from was growing. Farm-to-table restaurants and juice bars were just beginning to gain traction and buzz. Boutique fitness studios, devoted to just one type of workout, were emerging. And New Yorkers, post-recession, were looking for holistic practices and services much closer to home and easier on their wallets than trips to Bali, Thailand, or Canyon Ranch. So we did what we do best and wrote about it—all of it.

In those early days, we didn't necessarily have what you'd call a proper business plan, but we had a clear purpose and a pact—if, after six months, anyone was reading our writing (other than our well-intentioned friends and families), we'd build a real website and devote all of our time to making Well+Good our everything.

So we did. We tried workouts, credible nutrition concepts, every sound healthy approach attempting to fill in where Western life and lifestyle journalism left holes; we covered them all and we learned a lot. Workout studios filled up, beauty products sold out, and many of the experts we featured became household names.

Healthy living became a way of life and a way to connect with others. Instead of happy hour, people were grabbing a juice or "sweatworking" with colleagues. Culturally, we went from *Wait, what's almond butter?* to being able to buy it in every store. It all happened so fast. And we like to think we had a hand in that.

Now, 10 years later, the wellness world has exploded, both culturally and economically. Well+Good has grown to a staff of 60-plus supertalented people. And we reach an audience of more than 10 million people a month with our award-winning content.

Our mission has remained fairly unchanged: Well+Good is a trusted advisor for navigating the ever-expanding— and sometimes confusing—world of wellness. We define and demystify what it means to live a healthy life: breaking down both contemporary health practices and centuries-old traditions (yes, these can exist in harmony); calling *and* covering trends; and letting people know what to skip altogether.

But above all, we want your time on Well+Good, whether it's reading our daily articles, attending one of our in-person TALKS, joining us for a Well+Good Retreat, or even just scrolling through our Instagram feed, to be the best part of your day. We want to continue to transform lives and welcome people into the world of wellness in a way that works for them.

As a digital media company, we're especially excited to share this tangible book that you can leave out on your counter, splatter with food, and dog-ear to your heart's content. We always joke that you can't hug the internet—but you *can* hug this cookbook, which is filled with

OUR MISSION HAS REMAINED FAIRLY UNCHANGED: WELL+GOOD IS A TRUSTED ADVISOR FOR NAVIGATING THE EVER-EXPANDING— AND SOMETIMES CONFUSING—WORLD OF WELLNESS.

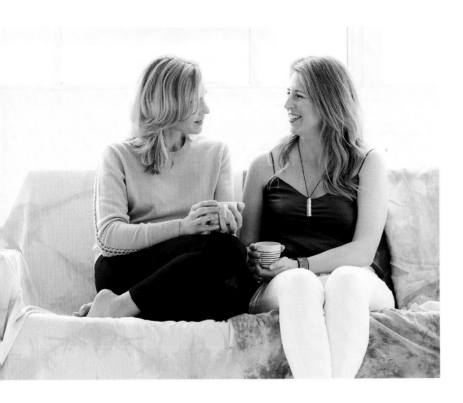

recipes from 100 of the healthiest people out there: wellness luminaries whom we respect, whose careers we've been covering for years, and who live crazy-busy lives, just like you do.

We tapped these wellness experts to share the recipes they've made at home 80 trillion times and will make a trillion more—these recipes are that good, and that easy. In this book, the experts have let us into their kitchens, and we're thrilled to earn a spot in yours. We owe a lot of gratitude to the people featured in this book, and to those who've worked tirelessly behind the scenes. It takes a village, and we're incredibly thankful to ours.

Tell us which recipes you make and become obsessed with! We're at @iamwellandgood and @wellandgoodeats on Instagram. Whether you've been with us since that first article, recently found us online, or just learned about us from this book, we're glad you're part of our community. And it makes us so happy to share our story and this cookbook with you.

*Alexia
+ Melisse*

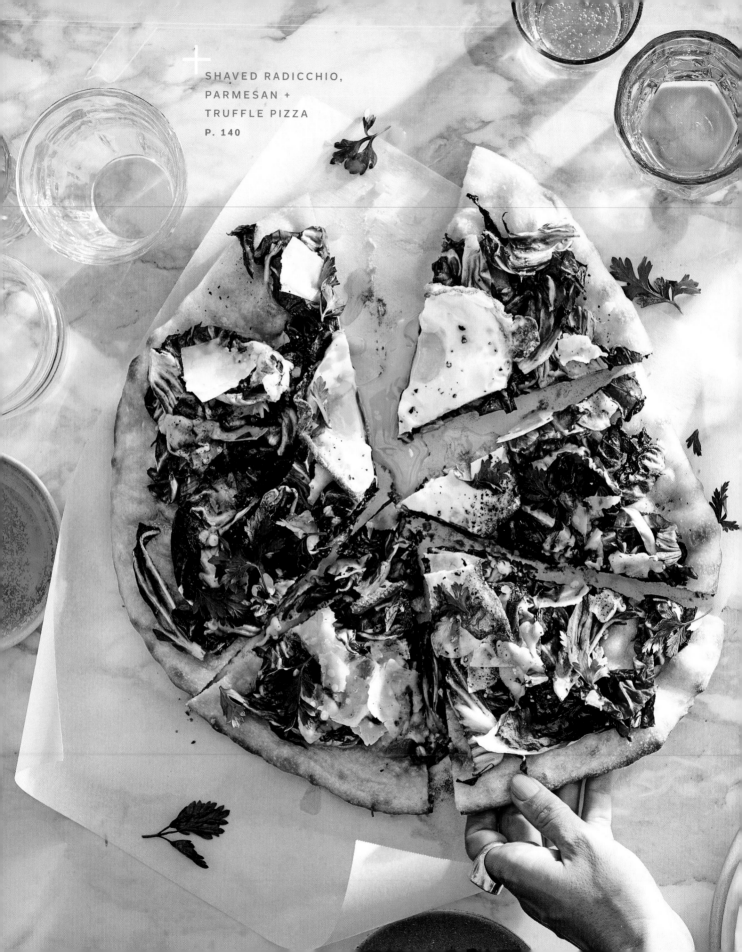

SHAVED RADICCHIO,
PARMESAN +
TRUFFLE PIZZA
P. 140

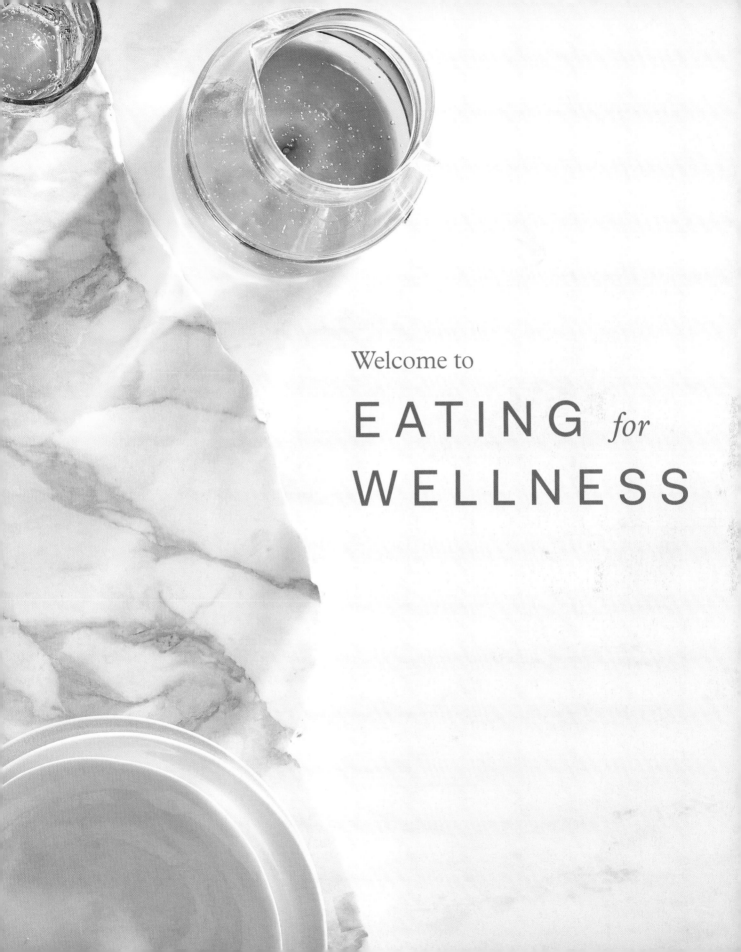

Welcome to

EATING *for* WELLNESS

ABOUT *this* BOOK

THIS BOOK IS ALL
ABOUT TAPPING THE
COLLECTIVE WISDOM
OF OUR GENIUS
HEALTHY COMMUNITY
FOR THEIR VERY
BEST RECIPES.

Well+Good has always covered the most interesting healthy food trends and nutrition intel, and shared the most delicious good-for-you recipes. We personally cook using recipes featured on Well+Good and send each other links to dishes we successfully make *a lot*. We're super digital, but we love cookbooks.

Making your own meals is one of the best ways to personalize your wellness, and yet, when life gets crazy it's often the first thing to go. But it doesn't have to be that way, and that's what you'll learn here. The kitchen is arguably where wellness starts (and sometimes ends). We've noticed a traffic pattern on Well+Good: *everyone* in our audience is looking for ways to eat healthy and quickly.

We were super hands-on, growing Well+Good organically, so we really got to know the movers and shakers at the very beginning of the wellness scene. We were discovering, interviewing, and often befriending first-generation founders—a stream of passionate entrepreneurs, charismatic instructors, and transformative integrative and functional medicine doctors. Some of these forces of nature have grown their businesses and scaled right alongside us, like Joey Gonzalez of Barry's

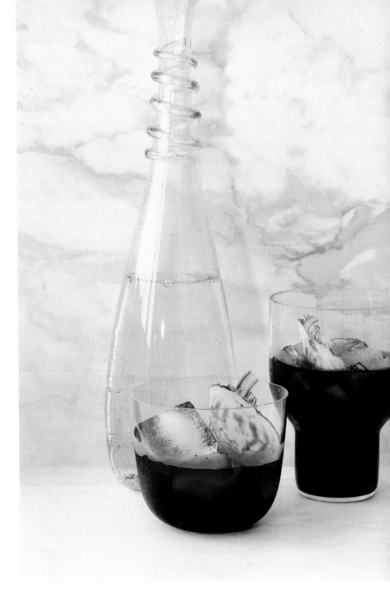

Bootcamp, Amanda Freeman of SLT, Dr. Frank Lipman, Whitney Tingle + Danielle DuBoise of Sakara Life, and modern spirituality maven Gabrielle Bernstein. They were shaping the wellness landscape and we helped shine a bright light on it, declaring a new era of wellness.

We've known and trusted these geniuses and their transformational work for a long time, which is why you'll find their recipes in this book. We've curated their go-to dishes and favorite easy meals—the ones they make over and over again for themselves, their families, their friends, and now for us. The *Well+Good* cookbook is all about tapping the collective wisdom of our genius healthy community for their very best recipes. And there are tricks, tips, and dishes we can apply to our own kitchens and recipe repertoires from theirs. This book serves up what our healthy community is cooking, with every recipe reflecting how the wellness world *really* eats.

We hand-selected each contributor, asking them how they channel Well+Good-ness in their kitchens on the day-to-day—and how we can do the same. We made a point to include contributors from across the wellness scene—so you'll not only find nutrition and fitness experts here, but also meditation, sleep, and hormone specialists. Learning that doughnuts can count as a post-workout snack (thanks for the tip, Karena Dawn + Katrina Scott), or how the lead dancer of the American Ballet Theater transforms flounder (we see you, Misty Copeland) can inspire a dish that just might never have occurred to you while you were pacing around the grocery store.

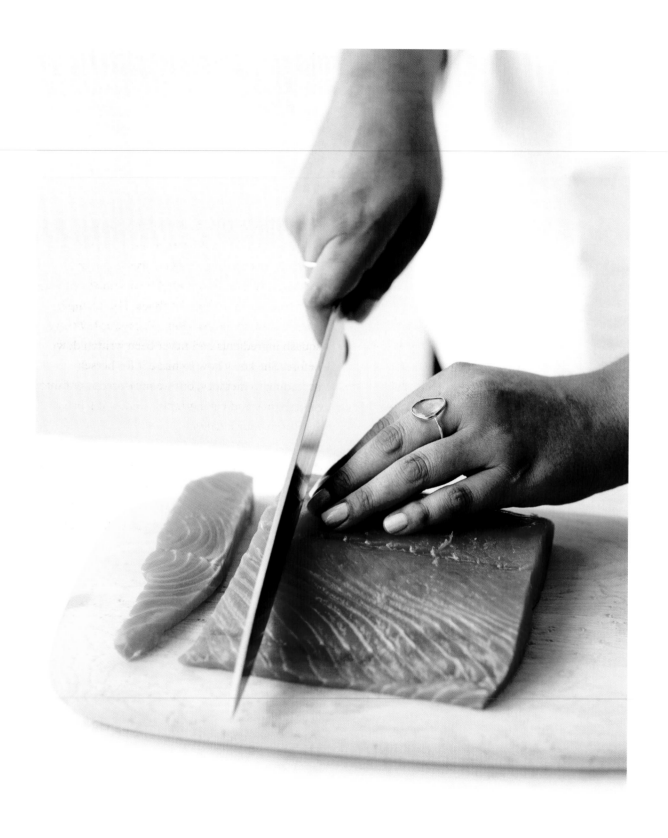

ABOUT *the* RECIPES

THESE RECIPES
ARE OPPORTUNITIES
TO BE WELL+GOOD
WHENEVER YOU EAT.

At its core, this book gives you more than 100 delicious dishes. We tested every one of them (frequently in tiny kitchens without much elbowroom, if that resonates), and sometimes even translated them for the cookbook. For example, fitness phenom Taryn Toomey's precise kabocha squash ingredients had never been written down before. She knew how to make it for herself according to memory, but we measured it out into tablespoons and baking times, so now it'll live forever in your kitchen.

Anything that tasted like blah "health food" didn't make the cut. We also said buh-bye to anything that didn't offer the ease we were looking for—the average recipe here takes fewer than 30 minutes from start to spoonful.

But these dishes aren't *just* great additions to your recipe repertoire. They're also opportunities to be Well+Good whenever you eat. Each offers you both health and wellness. What's the difference? Well, there isn't really one, but the following pages outline what we mean. . . .

No matter your dietary preferences or nutritional style, we have healthy recipes here that will work for you. These include:

DAIRY-FREE: This means no animal-derived milk, cheese, yogurt, cottage cheese, sour cream, ice cream, whey, or whey proteins. Some people choose to avoid casein, a protein, or lactose, a sugar that can cause digestive woes or inflammation, while others may be allergic.

GLUTEN-FREE: For many people it's not about going low-carb; rather, it's about dodging the gluten proteins found in wheat, rye, barley, bulgur, and couscous, which can cause an allergic, inflammatory response. Celiacs have the most extreme, sometimes life-threatening sensitivity, and don't have the capacity to digest gluten.

KETOGENIC: The keto diet is centered around producing ketones in the body through fasting and food choices so that fat is used as the main energy source, as opposed to carbs. The diet is high in fats (90 to 100 grams a day) and veggies, is low-carb (fewer than 30 grams a day), and includes adequate protein.

LOW-FODMAP: FODMAP is an acronym for six different groups of short-chain carbohydrates, all of which are said to be poorly absorbed and can cause bloating for people with sensitive digestive systems: fructose (simple sugar often found in fruit), lactose, fructans (found in many gluten-based grains), galactans (found in legumes), and polyols (a sugar alcohol). A low-FODMAP diet avoids any food with carbohydrates from these six subgroups.

LOW-INFLAMMATION: A low-inflammation diet limits any foods directly linked to causing inflammation: anything processed, high in sugar, or made with refined foods. Gluten and dairy can also be inflammatory. Instead, a low-inflammation diet centers around eating whole, nutrient-rich foods such as leafy greens, healthy fats, fermented foods, and inflammation-fighting spices, such as turmeric and ginger.

PALEO: Paleo eaters aim to eat the way our ancestors may have eaten, before processed foods and the food industries behind them became mainstays. They favor high-nutrient, whole foods, including grass-fed meat, sustainable seafood, lots of vegetables, fruit, seeds, and nuts. Dairy, grains, and legumes are all off the table.

VEGAN: Vegans don't eat any form of animal products, including eggs, dairy, and honey. Often, the term "vegan" extends beyond dietary preferences, and is one of many lifestyle choices based on the health of the environment and animals. Many people who subscribe to this nutritional philosophy may also refer to themselves as "plant-based."

VEGETARIAN: Vegetarians don't eat meat, but unlike vegans they may eat eggs, dairy, honey, and in some cases fish (though technically eating the latter would make them pescatarian).

In addition to these health factors, we've also ensured these recipes will help you get specific about the wellness benefits of your food. These include eating for:

BETTER DIGESTION: It's all about keeping your belly happy. Get great gut health by including fermented foods, getting your daily dose of probiotics, and avoiding added sugar and processed foods.

BETTER ENERGY: Go for lots of fruits and veggies (especially berries and leafy greens), switch to whole-food carbs like sweet potatoes, and make sure you're getting your Recommended Daily Allowance of B vitamins.

BETTER FOCUS: Boost your brain health by getting lots of omega-3s on your plate (hope you like salmon, sardines, and extra-virgin olive oil), as well as eggs, leafy greens, and dark chocolate.

BETTER MOOD: Get a handle on your blood sugar by avoiding skipping meals, eating mood-stabilizing good fats (hello, avocados), and boosting your intake of foods rich in vitamin B, D, and K, like grass-fed beef, spinach, and chickpeas.

BETTER SEX: Yes, what you've heard about oysters is true. But don't forget all the other foods that can rev your engine: everything from broccoli and pistachios to chia seeds.

BETTER SKIN: Healthy fats are your friend—as are fiber, foods rich in vitamins A and C (hey there, daily greens), and hydrating foods like cucumber and watermelon.

BETTER SLEEP: Timing is everything here. (As in, not eating big meals or drinking alcohol before bedtime.) Instead, boosting your magnesium and calcium intake and sipping melatonin-boosting tart cherry juice can help transform bedtime.

Peppered throughout the book are go-deep guides on what eating for wellness really means. They're written by super-credentialed Well+Good Council members and experts and provide extra intel on how food can help you get to how you want to feel.

Our curated recipe collection will help you with all of these health and wellness factors—and overall, leave you feeling really good about the choices you're making at mealtime. We think it's more important (and, frankly, more interesting) to focus on the nutrition of ingredients and what food can offer us, rather than getting hung up on calorie and carb count. This cookbook, and the Well+Good ethos that runs through it, is based on functional nutrition and informed by experts—not by wellness BS. We've made it as easy as possible for your meals to serve *you*.

HOW *to* USE THIS BOOK

Our recipes are organized in a mostly traditional manner—or at least, how we know our Well+Good reader likes to eat: Yes, we appreciate a sit-down meal, but sometimes we kind of love to graze all day long. **Morning Meals** are for energizing first thing. Some can be prepped ahead because we know how hard it can be to get it together when you're in a rush. **Smoothies + Smoothie Bowls** earned their own chapter because we like to enjoy them at any and every time of day. **Light Fare** is what you need when you're looking for something simple—but don't be fooled! These meals are all nutrient-dense and stand on their own or can be added to a main for an effortless multi-course meal.

WE HAVE SIMPLE
SOLUTIONS FOR
HEALTHY DISHES
YOU NEVER THOUGHT
YOU COULD
MAKE YOURSELF.

Mains are meant to be shared and as a bonus, can often be meal-prepped. We have weeknight staples to work into your regular routine, updated versions of classics, and even simple solutions for healthy dishes you never thought you could make yourself. We paired **Sweets + Snacks** together because our desserts are *not* sugar bombs and many of our snacks are exciting enough to fuel a workout or end a meal. Lastly, the final section of **Drinks** is not just for cocktail hour—these are turbo-charged coffees, tonics, and OK, fine, a nightcap or two.

On each recipe page, you'll find which expert contributed it, and in the headnote, insider intel on how they came up with the recipe, when or why they like to make it, and a little bit about their own eating preferences, too. Read these—pretty please! You'll pick up tips and tricks, and also become more intimately familiar with the OGs of wellness. And if an ingredient is a little bit specialty, that's how you'll know where to find it.

Also on each page is a list of every health and wellness factor that a recipe has to offer you. So when you're thumbing through, you can find what works best for exactly how you want to eat. If you are looking to go a little deeper into the health and wellness aspects of your meals, though, we've got that covered, too. On page 260, you'll find an index where each recipe is categorized both in terms of which healthy eating preference it fits into, and what its wellness benefit is. On a dairy-free kick? Take your pick from the recipes that exclude it. If you have a big meeting tomorrow, for tonight we suggest a dinner that gives you better focus. Whichever way you choose to use this book, we've made sure it will work for you.

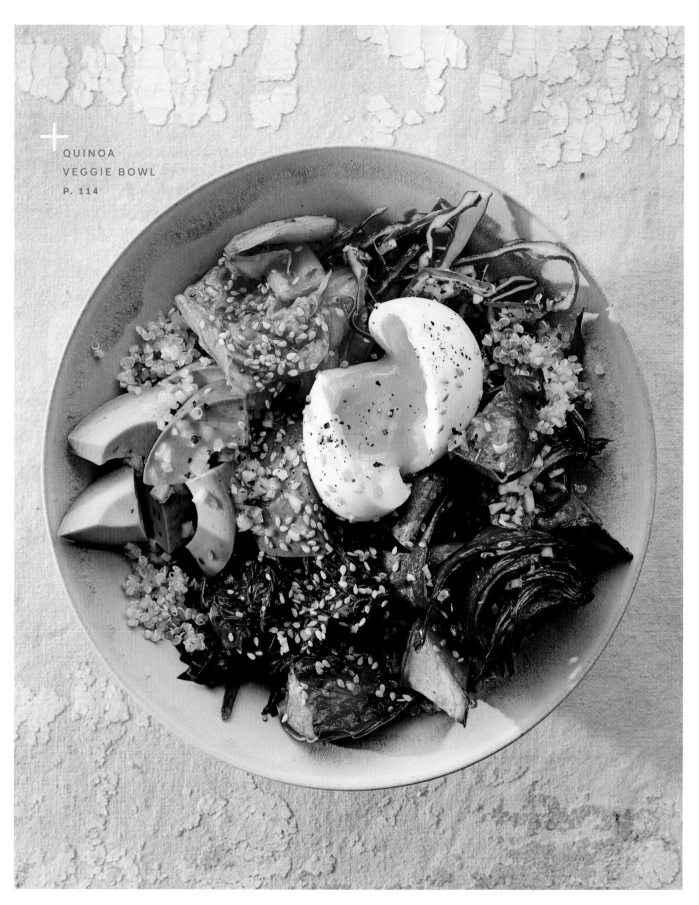

QUINOA
VEGGIE BOWL
P. 114

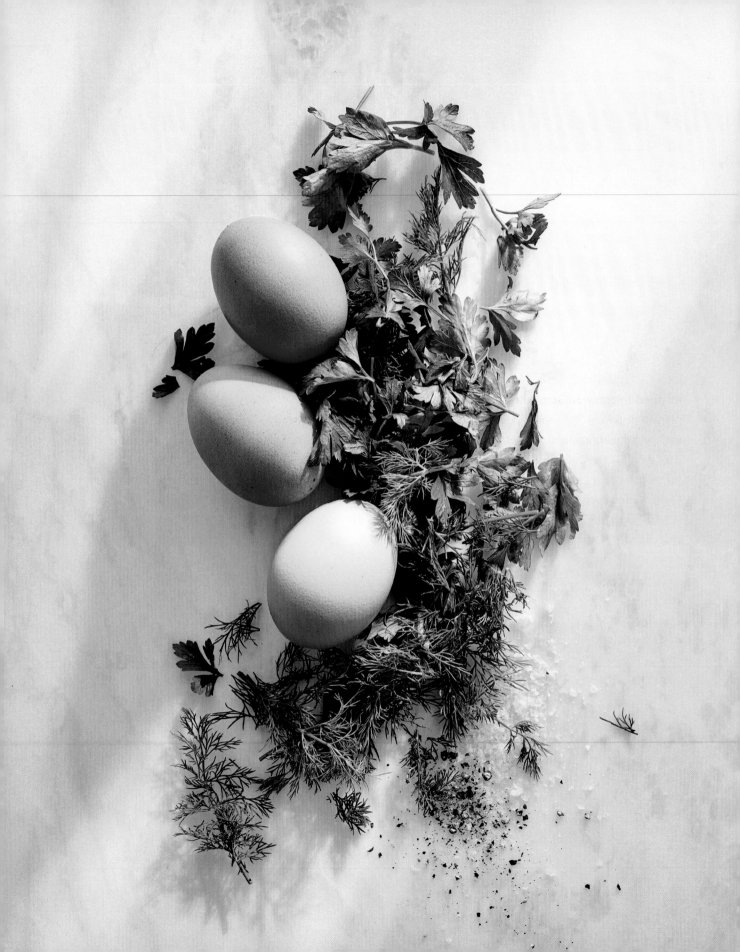

WELL+GOOD INGREDIENTS

Grocery stores nationwide are stocking up their health-food staples, superfoods, and organic sections. If you don't see something you're looking for, just ask—sometimes they're more inspired to carry an item when they know you plan to purchase it. Whole Foods, Trader Joe's, and your local farmers' market are still your best bets for produce and not-yet-mainstream ingredients or pantry staples made by smaller brands. However, we love two amazing online resources that will get you non-perishable groceries by mail: Thrive Market and Brandless.

Eating for wellness is not about making yourself crazy trying to restock your whole kitchen. As we already mentioned, when a recipe includes a rarer ingredient, the headnote or tip will tell you where to find it. But these are some ingredients we thought warranted a few more words.

ADAPTOGENS: We wrote this book to be for everyone. Maybe there's no room in your shopping cart for you to be buying schisandra berries, or maybe you're allergic to the idea of mushroom powder. We offer substitutes within the recipes and made sure they taste delicious and are nourishing either way. If you're using them, though, please do so knowing some of these plants are in the supplements family, so check if they work for you if you're pregnant or have other health considerations.

CACAO: Cacao is very different than cocoa powder, which contains milk, sugar, and lots of other additives and fillers. Real, raw cacao powder is made from ground cacao beans—and nothing else. Because of this, it costs a bit more, but in this form chocolate's really a good-for-you food: It's high in fiber, magnesium, and even protein. You can find it in the smoothie superfood aisle or online.

COOKING OIL: Extra-virgin olive oil, coconut oil, ghee, and grass-fed butter are all fair game in this book. Sometimes the choice is about dietary preference (i.e., avoiding dairy or lactose) and other times it's about the oil's smoking point. EVOO has the lowest of these, so some people prefer not to use it at high heat where its nutrients are lost. But all of these oils have health benefits and are considered a source of good fats.

DAIRY: Vegans and Paleos may deliberately avoid it, as will the lactose intolerant, but a lot of people really love it. We've gone light on the dairy in this cookbook, but as personal fans of yogurt, some recipes with dairy ingredients do appear here. For those of you who don't eat dairy, plenty of non-dairy alternatives are available in supermarkets, including substitutions for milk (from almost every kind of nut!) and cheese. Some nut milks, like the kind in shelf-stable cartons, are often diluted (read: less flavorful) and contain fillers, emulsifiers, and a lot of sugar; look for ones with only a few ingredients listed, and choose the unsweetened varieties. If you're a DIYer, try making them yourself.

FLOUR (ALMOND FLOUR, ARROWROOT FLOUR, COCONUT FLOUR, OAT FLOUR, RICE FLOUR, AND TAPIOCA FLOUR): The wellness community has flocked to gluten-free flours, which handle a bit differently than the all-purpose, wheat-derived varieties. If you follow the recipes closely in this book, you'll be fine. Almond flour, for example, is just finely milled nuts, so it adds moisture and protein to baking—and it's actually not that hard to make yourself. All of these flours are widely available online. We love Bob's Red Mill, but there are plenty of great brands out there.

SALT: Some say that Himalayan sea salt has more nutrients than plain old table salt or iodized salt—that it includes trace minerals like calcium and magnesium—so why not add it to your meals. Many seem to be fans of its coarser texture. (You can buy pink Himalayan sea salt in an unrefined form to grind with each use or in a fine pre-ground form.) Same goes for kosher salt, which also has a larger crystal size, and has a particular appeal among chefs. Each recipe specifies which type its contributor prefers to use.

SUGAR: We mostly stay away from refined white granulated sugar in this book. Instead, many of the recipes use naturally sweet foods, like bananas or dates, or monk fruit sweetener. (Monk fruit sweetener has the closest taste to sugar—in fact, it is very, very sweet—and is heat stable, meaning it's good for cooking and baking.) In general, refined sugar sneaks into a lot of foods you'd be surprised to find it in, like store-bought bread and yogurt, which is probably why most of us surpass the daily recommended amount of 25 grams way too easily. Read labels closely, especially those of nut milks and nut butters. Reach for the unsweetened varieties, and avoid anything labeled low-fat or fat-free, which usually contains a lot of sugar.

When to Go Organic

We don't expect you to be 100 percent organic 100 percent of the time (we're not). Until the cost of and access to these foods improves, we treat buying organic as more of a preference. That said, there are few foods for which we strongly recommend holding out for organic: corn (unless you know the farm stand), soy, and canola— since those crops are some of the most genetically modified and sprayed. The Environmental Working Group's Dirty Dozen—and growing—list shares intel on which produce has high pesticide use (so you should buy it organic, when possible) or where you can save a few bucks and buy the regular stuff (mostly what you peel). For meat and eggs, go for grass-fed and free-range poultry when possible. If you know a butcher or farmer who'll tell you the source and care of the produce and animals, even better. Same with dairy—go with organic or a brand that shares its sourcing information.

A FINAL NOTE

Here's the thing: We're not doctors (though some star in this book), but hope you'll feel better following the Well+Good cooking ethos.

Healthy eating is so not about a deprivation dinner-plate of salads and chicken breasts—please memorize that. There's a world of nutrient-dense, great-for-you foods out there awaiting a spot at your table.

Food is tasty fuel and can be thoughtfully used to your advantage—it can also be incredibly delish and super fun. It's okay to turn slices of sweet potato into toast and put blue spirulina powder in your smoothie bowl because it looks cool. Your body won't mind a bit, because it feels good, too.

We're also not chefs (but we feature plenty of them here, too). As the master of your own menu every day, you have our total permission to taste along the way, swap in (or out whatever you like, and when in doubt, roughly chop! No wizardry is required when you eat for wellness.

NOW LET'S GET STARTED.

MORNING
MEALS

Supermodel and Well+Good Council member Elle Macpherson is famously sporty; you're much more likely to find her on a surfboard than a treadmill. She takes a similarly *joie de vivre* approach to nutrition, with an emphasis on organic, seasonal whole foods, whipped up into something delicious. "For me, it is about living every day as clean, green, and active as I can," says the cofounder of WelleCo, a line of plant-based elixirs and supplements available in their online shop and in stores throughout the world. Blend this recipe early in the week for a nutrient-dense dessert-like breakfast that's ready to eat whenever you are.

CHOCOLATE MOUSSE
WITH FRESH RASPBERRIES + CACAO NIBS

Serves 3 or 4

3 cups mashed avocado
(from 4 to 5 small avocados)

¼ cup coconut oil

1 tablespoon vanilla powder
or extract

¼ cup almond butter

¾ cup pure maple syrup

1½ cups raw cacao powder

¼ cup cold filtered water

3 tablespoons chocolate protein
powder

Pinch of flaky sea salt

Fresh raspberries, for topping
(optional)

Cacao nibs, for topping (optional)

+

DAIRY-FREE

GLUTEN-FREE

KETOGENIC

LOW-INFLAMMATION

VEGAN

VEGETARIAN

BETTER ENERGY

BETTER SKIN

1. In a food processor or blender, combine the avocado, coconut oil, and vanilla. Blend until smooth, about 2 minutes.

2. Add the almond butter, maple syrup, cacao powder, filtered water, protein powder, and salt. Blend until thoroughly combined.

3. Scrape the mousse into three or four individual bowls and top with fresh raspberries and cacao nibs, as desired. Cover any leftovers with plastic wrap; they'll keep in the refrigerator for up to 1 week.

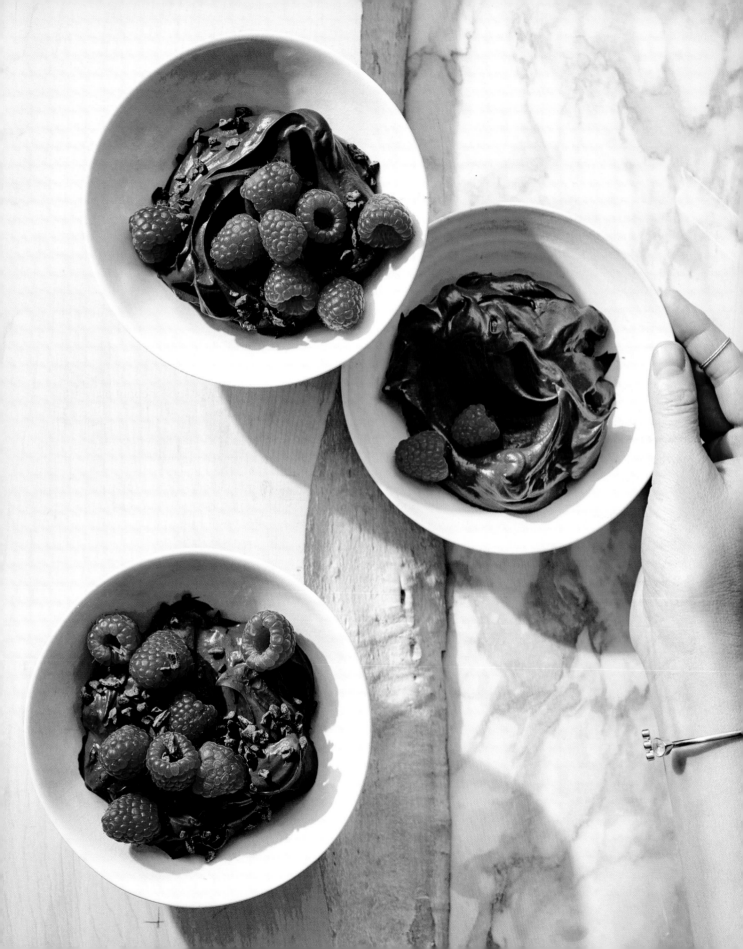

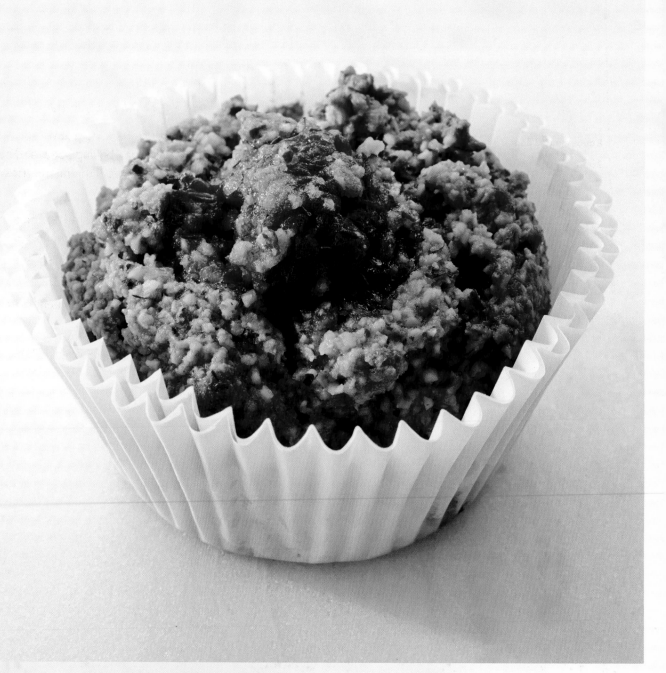

Jenny Carr created this recipe on her personal-turned-professional path to healing chronic health conditions with anti-inflammatory foods, which are less likely to trigger allergies or digestive issues. "These gluten-free muffins are the perfect breakfast on a cozy day at home," says the expert, mom-preneur, and best-selling author of *Peace of Cake: The Secret to an Anti-Inflammatory Diet.* Eat these muffins—bursting with flavor and the perfect touch of sweetness from honey (*not* the refined granular stuff)—knowing you are receiving a solid dose of anti-inflammatory goodness, and plan to bake them on repeat.

RASPBERRY-ALMOND MUFFINS

Makes 12 muffins

2 cups almond flour

2 large eggs

¼ cup coconut oil, melted

¼ cup honey

1 tablespoon pure vanilla extract

½ teaspoon almond extract

1 teaspoon apple cider vinegar

½ teaspoon baking soda

¼ teaspoon sea salt

1 cup fresh or strained thawed frozen raspberries

1. Preheat the oven to 350°F. Line a muffin tin with paper liners.

2. In a medium bowl, whisk together the almond flour, eggs, melted coconut oil, honey, vanilla, almond extract, vinegar, baking soda, and salt until thoroughly combined. Using a spatula, gently fold the raspberries into the batter.

3. Using a ¼-cup measure, drop the batter into the prepared muffin cups. Bake for 15 minutes, then rotate the pan and bake for 15 minutes more, or until the edges are golden, the muffins are firm in the center, and a tester inserted into the center of a muffin comes out clean.

4. Remove the pan from the oven. Let the muffins cool in the pan for at least 15 minutes before removing from the pan.

5. Serve, or transfer to an airtight container, cover with a paper towel and the container lid, and store at room temperature for 1 to 2 days.

+

DAIRY-FREE

GLUTEN-FREE

LOW-INFLAMMATION

PALEO

VEGETARIAN

BETTER SKIN

Global fitness star Emily Skye is proof that Australia tends to take the cake (well, in this case, the pancake) when it comes to leading the wellness scene. The fitness model and trainer shares her real-life eating routine with millions of social followers through FIT (Fitness Inspiration Transformation), the nutrition and workout program she founded. And with these low-glycemic, gluten-free pancakes, Emily turns the lazy-Sunday-morning go-to into a daily option, with enough protein—about 30 grams!—to refuel your muscles after an early-morning sweat session.

APPLE + CINNAMON PANCAKES

Makes 4 pancakes

1 medium apple, peeled, cored, and shredded (about ¾ cup)

⅓ cup almond meal or almond flour

1 large egg

1 egg white

⅓ cup plain protein powder

½ teaspoon ground cinnamon, plus more for serving

Unsweetened almond milk, if needed

1 to 2 tablespoons coconut oil, for cooking

1½ tablespoons yogurt, for serving

1. Put the shredded apple in a clean kitchen towel and squeeze over the sink to remove the excess liquid. Transfer the apple to a medium bowl. Add the almond meal, egg, egg white, protein powder, and cinnamon and stir to evenly combine. If the mixture seems too dry, add a splash of almond milk.

2. Melt 1 tablespoon coconut oil in a large skillet over medium heat. When it shimmers, working in batches, use a ¼-cup measure to generously scoop the mixture into the pan to form 4 pancakes. Use a spatula to flatten the pancakes. Cook for 2 to 3 minutes, until bubbles appear on top. Flip the pancakes and cook on the other side for 2 to 3 minutes more, until lightly brown on the bottom. Transfer to a plate and repeat with the remaining batter.

3. Serve warm, topped with the yogurt and a sprinkle of cinnamon.

GLUTEN-FREE

VEGETARIAN

BETTER SKIN

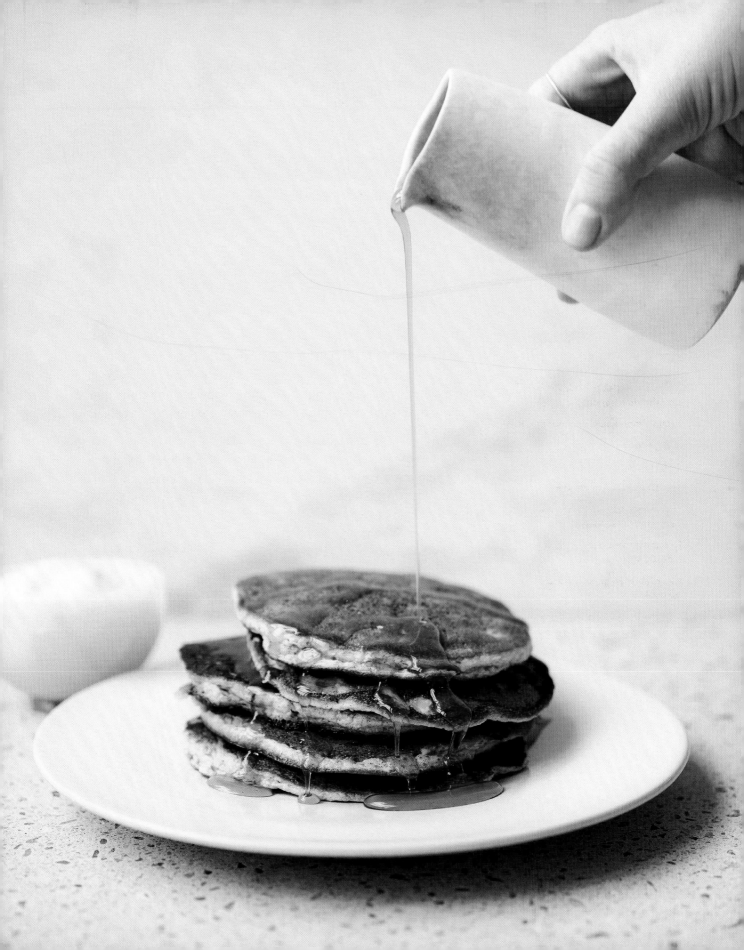

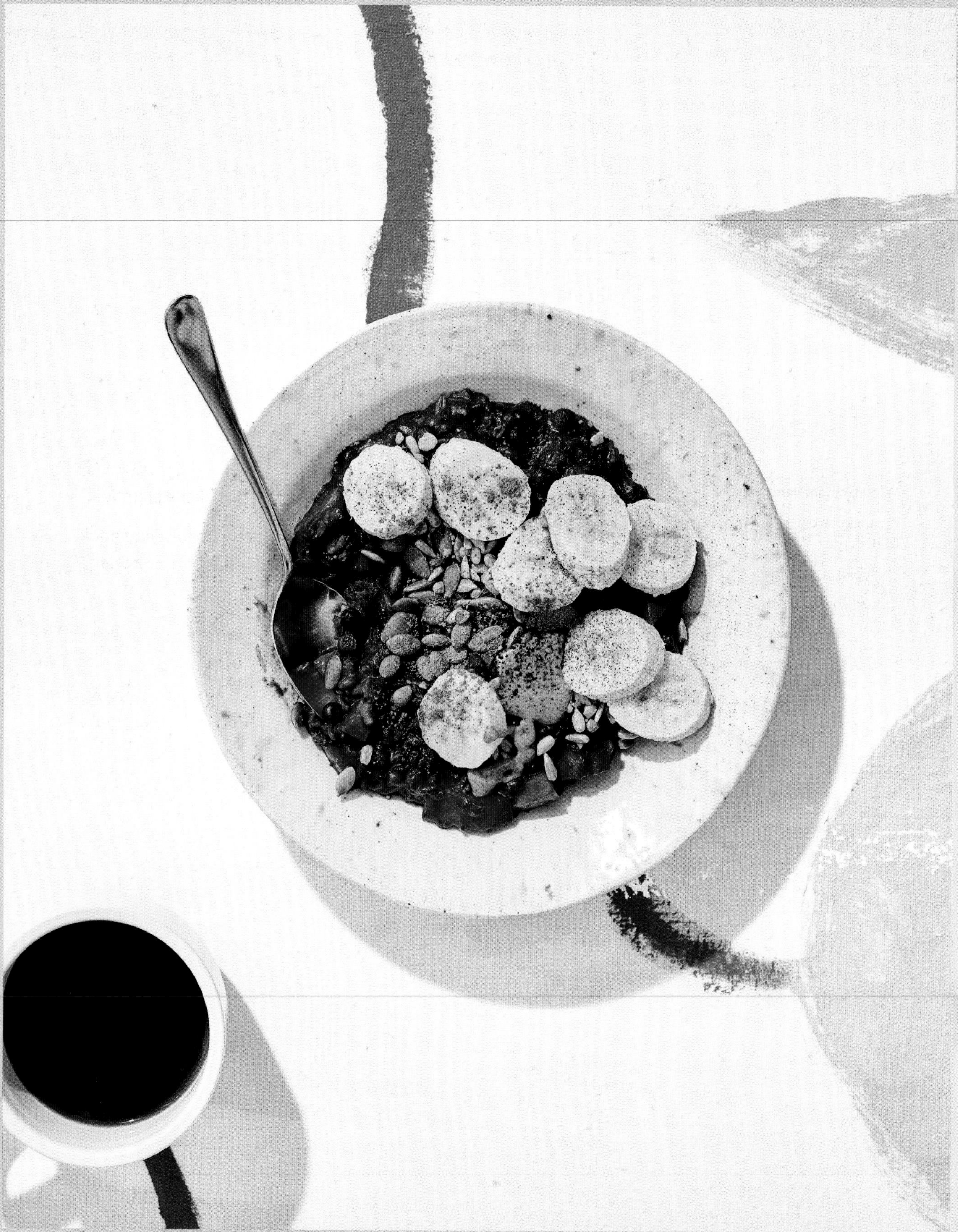

KSENIA
AVDULOVA

As the #bowlgoals guru behind the popular *Breakfast Criminals* blog, Ksenia Avdulova believes that how you start your day is how you live your life. "The practice of intention-setting is my favorite morning ritual," says the healthy-breakfast obsessive and creator of photogenic food. "*How* we eat is just as important as what's on our plate." Packed with digestion-boosting enzymes and topped with moringa, an anti-inflammatory powerhouse, this recipe is also a sentimental favorite for Ksenia, since it's inspired by the blueberry oatmeal her mother fed her as a child whenever she had a cold. You can find moringa leaf powder in the supermarket superfood aisle and online.

SUPERFOOD GALAXY OATMEAL

Serves 1

½ cup instant oats

1 cup fresh or thawed frozen blueberries

½ apple, cored and diced

⅓ cup unsweetened almond milk

1 teaspoon ground cinnamon

1 teaspoon preserves, honey, or brown rice syrup

OPTIONAL TOPPINGS

1 teaspoon pumpkin seed butter

2 tablespoons raw pumpkin seeds

2 tablespoons raw sunflower seeds

1 teaspoon moringa leaf powder

1 banana, sliced

1. In a medium saucepan, combine the oats and 1 cup water and bring to a boil over high heat. Reduce the heat to medium and cook, stirring occasionally, for 5 minutes, or until the mixture thickens slightly.

2. Add the blueberries and apple, reduce the heat to low, and cook, stirring occasionally, for 5 minutes, or until the blueberries soften. Gently mash the blueberries with a spoon to color the oatmeal purple.

3. Stir in the almond milk and add the cinnamon. Cook until the oatmeal thickens further, about 3 minutes more.

4. Transfer the oatmeal to a bowl and stir in the preserves. Top with the pumpkin seed butter, pumpkin seeds, sunflower seeds, moringa, and banana as desired, and enjoy.

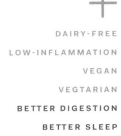

DAIRY-FREE

LOW-INFLAMMATION

VEGAN

VEGTARIAN

BETTER DIGESTION

BETTER SLEEP

KARENA
DAWN
+
KATRINA
SCOTT

"Doughnuts are my favorite, and I've been obsessed with matcha lately, so these are the ultimate treat for me," says Katrina Scott, who, with Karena Dawn, cofounded Tone It Up—an online fitness community whose 1 million-plus members are seriously passionate about getting results (and encouraging each other). So, doughnuts as a post-workout snack? It wouldn't seem like an obvious pick for the Tone It Up crew, but these protein powder–packed creations are closer to homemade energy bars than Krispy Kremes. And with an anti-inflammatory kick of matcha, these delicious treats are definitely trainer-approved—which definitely justifies owning a doughnut pan.

HONEY-MATCHA–GLAZED DOUGHNUTS

Makes 6 to 8 doughnuts

FOR THE DOUGHNUTS

Coconut oil spray

½ cup unflavored pea
protein powder

¼ cup gluten-free oat flour

¼ cup almond flour

1 teaspoon baking powder

½ teaspoon ground cinnamon

¼ teaspoon sea salt

¼ cup unsweetened almond milk

¼ cup pure maple syrup

1 large egg

1 teaspoon pure vanilla extract

1 tablespoon coconut oil, melted

FOR THE GLAZE

¼ cup wildflower honey

1 teaspoon matcha green tea powder,
plus more for topping

Sliced almonds, for topping (optional)

1. Make the doughnuts. Preheat the oven to 350°F. Spray a doughnut pan with coconut oil spray.

2. In a medium bowl, whisk together the protein powder, oat flour, almond flour, baking powder, cinnamon, and salt until thoroughly combined.

3. In a separate medium bowl, combine the almond milk, maple syrup, egg, vanilla, and melted coconut oil. Whisk thoroughly to combine.

4. Add the wet ingredients to the dry ingredients and whisk to combine.

5. Pour the batter into the prepared pan. Bake for 15 to 20 minutes, or until a tester inserted into one or two doughnuts comes out clean. Remove from the oven and let cool completely in the pan.

6. Meanwhile, make the glaze. In a medium bowl, whisk together the honey and matcha.

7. When the doughnuts have cooled, one at a time, dip their tops into the glaze, letting any excess drip off the sides. Set the glazed doughnuts on a plate or wire rack and sprinkle with additional matcha and the almonds, if desired. Let the glaze set completely before serving or storing.

8. Store in an airtight container at room temperature for up to 1 day.

DAIRY-FREE

GLUTEN-FREE

LOW-INFLAMMATION

VEGETARIAN

BETTER FOCUS

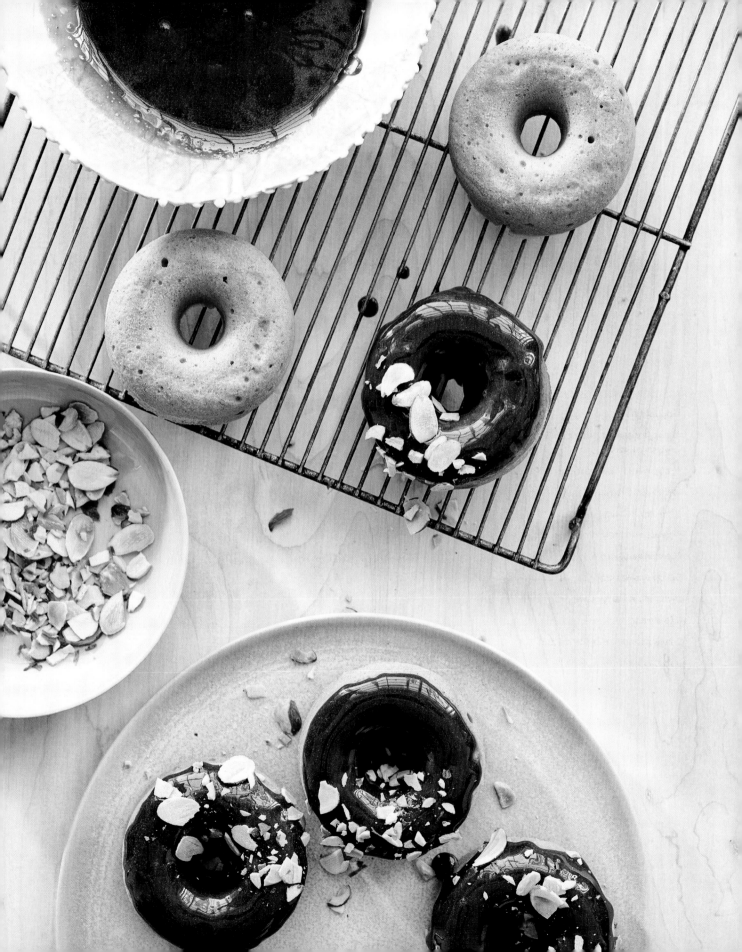

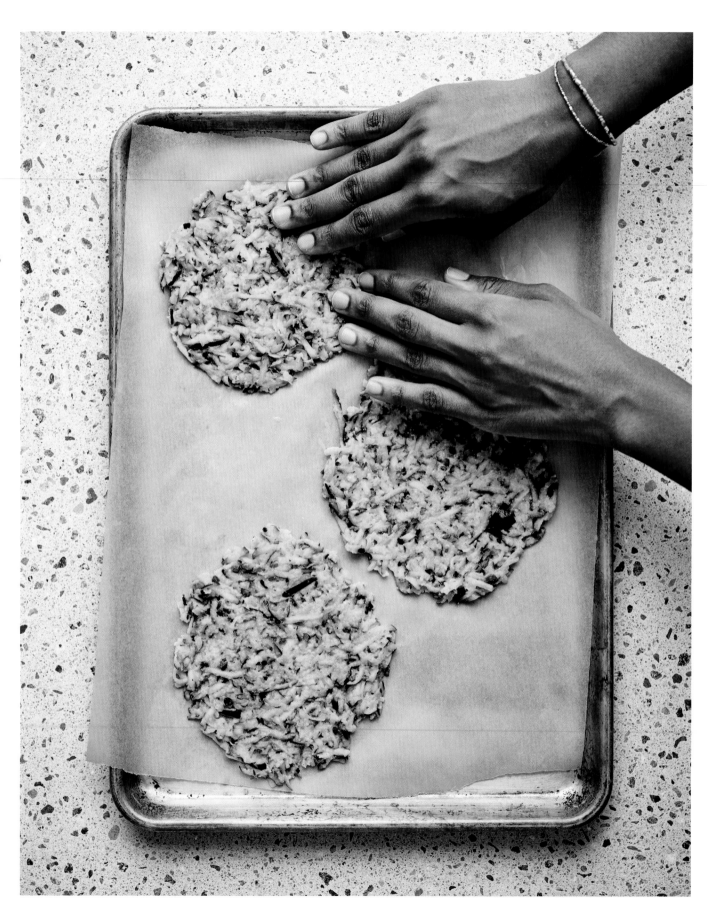

Mark Sisson doesn't deal in regret or restriction. "I center my eating around healthy, nutrient-dense food like meats and vegetables every day—but I won't deny myself if there's something I'd like to enjoy on occasion," says the Paleo OG, who, as the founder of Mark's Daily Apple and Primal Kitchen, has helped turbocharge the eating philosophy's growth. Instead of ignoring his crepe cravings, Mark created this lighter, zucchini-and-thyme-based alternative to the traditionally gluten-heavy wraps. Fill with smoked salmon and chives, or stack a few on a plate to top with a dollop of nut-milk yogurt.

SAVORY ZUCCHINI + THYME CREPES

Makes 4 crepes

3 cups grated zucchini
(from about 1 pound zucchini)

1 large egg, beaten

2 teaspoons avocado oil or
extra-virgin olive oil

1 garlic clove, finely chopped

Leaves from 4 or 5 sprigs thyme

1 tablespoon coconut flour

2 teaspoons tapioca flour

¼ teaspoon kosher salt

Pinch of freshly ground
black pepper

Fillings of your choice, if desired

1. Preheat the oven to 450°F. Line a large baking sheet with parchment paper.

2. Working in batches, wrap the grated zucchini in a thin kitchen towel and squeeze repeatedly over the sink to remove as much moisture as possible.

3. In a large bowl, whisk together the egg, avocado oil, garlic, thyme, coconut flour, tapioca flour, salt, and pepper until smooth, with no lumps remaining. Add the zucchini and mix with a spoon until completely combined.

4. Scoop about ⅓ cup of the zucchini mixture onto the prepared baking sheet. Use your fingers to press the mixture into a 6-inch circle, about ¼ inch thick. Repeat to make a total of 4 crepes, spacing them evenly on the baking sheet. Bake for about 20 minutes, or until lightly browned around the edges.

5. Remove the pan from the oven. Let the crepes sit on the pan until cool to the touch, then carefully peel them off the parchment paper.

6. Fill the crepes with scrambled eggs, smoked salmon, fresh chives, nut-milk yogurt, or anything else you like. Zucchini crepes taste best if eaten soon after they are made.

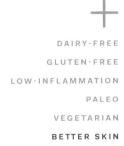

DAIRY-FREE

GLUTEN-FREE

LOW-INFLAMMATION

PALEO

VEGETARIAN

BETTER SKIN

EAT FOR BETTER SKIN

It wasn't long ago that dermatologists believed the food we ate had little—if any—connection to skincare issues like acne, hyperpigmentation, or even a basic lack of glow. Studies have since recognized that sugar, trans fats, and processed foods are bad for your health in general, and are also not great for your largest organ: your skin. In particular, researchers have called out how inflammatory foods like dairy and sugar can—and often do—cause issues such as acne and glycation, a process that may affect skin luminosity and harm bouncy-skin proteins, like collagen.

But aren't skincare products also very responsible for amazing skin? Yes, beauty products are key, but it's not just about the bottles and tubes we buy. You can't rub on great skincare products expecting them to do all the work. Sorry. Great skin is a reflection of health on a deeper level— your gut health, the nutrient quality of your food choices, and how you deal with stress.

While dermatologists have started to encourage us to step slowly away from French fries, pizza, and ice cream, you're still not super likely to get a grocery list for great skin at your doctor's office. And that's okay, because we'll give you one here.

My beauty-food recommendations are pretty simple. They come from working with countless clients and celebrities, and from healing my own skin woes. My biggest, most helpful tip is probably this: When people eat more plants or a plant-based diet, their skin really benefits. (I've personally been all plant-based for over twelve years.) The Mayo Clinic also zeroes in on greens, seeds, nuts, and legumes as "skin-friendly foods." Plant foods contain complex phytonutrients, including vitamins, minerals, fiber, and enzymes. They help create a lit-from-within condition for naturally healthy skin, while inflammatory foods may roadblock you.

> YOU CAN'T RUB ON GREAT SKINCARE PRODUCTS EXPECTING THEM TO DO ALL THE WORK. SORRY.

Here are my beauty foods and advice that can help give you the healthy, deep glow of amazing skin.

DEVELOP EXCELLENT DIGESTION.
Research now confirms a gut-brain-skin link, showing that a healthy gut microbiome can help with inflammation and oxidative stress (both of which play a role in accelerating skin aging), and may even help such conditions as acne and rosacea. Take probiotics (I recommend soil-based-organisms, or SBOs); eat plants that stimulate healthy digestion, like fennel, cilantro, and papaya; and incorporate fermented foods like sauerkraut, kombucha, and miso.

DRINK A LOW-SUGAR GREEN SMOOTHIE EVERY DAY. Years ago I created the Glowing Green Smoothie at my Los Angeles juice bar, Glow Bio, which has become my signature and daily go-to. It's loaded with nutrients that help detoxify and support glowing skin and sustained energy. I encourage you to mix and match greens and fruit in a daily smoothie, but stick with a ratio of around 70 percent greens to 30 percent high-fiber fruit, and add a good squeeze of lemon juice.

EAT FIBER. Fiber is key for gorgeous skin from a nutrition standpoint and because it helps keep everything moving through the digestive system. Reach for leafy greens like kale, beans and legumes, chia seeds, apples, and raspberries.

INCORPORATE AMAZING SKIN FOODS INTO YOUR MEALS. The following have proven compounds to support healthy skin:

+ Foods with high amounts of vitamin A and C: Dark leafy greens, carrots, beets, broccoli, and citrus fruit like grapefruit can help stimulate collagen synthesis and offer antioxidant support (which we need to help fend off damage caused by UV rays).

+ Anti-inflammatories: Turmeric is the front-runner, supported by studies, but foods like blueberries, moringa, spirulina, and chaga mushrooms are considered inflammation-fighting superfoods.

+ Hydrating foods like cucumber, watermelon, and coconut water (just watch the sugar).

+ Healthy fats like essential fatty acids from avocado and pumpkin seeds and gamma linoleic acid from seaweed help deeply nourish and rejuvenate skin. Don't skip these good fats; if you do, it'll show.

+ Beauty minerals help support cellular function: Bananas, cauliflower, sweet potatoes, nuts, seeds, and leafy greens like spinach are filled with beautifying minerals like calcium, zinc, biotin, iron, and potassium.

—KIMBERLY SNYDER, CN

Imagine if cardio, strength training, and Pilates had a baby—it would definitely be the SLT workout created by Amanda Freeman, who founded this super-smart fifty-minute class in 2011 and has since turned it into a national fitness chain. So, yes, her days are *packed*. Amanda preps these oats before she goes to sleep so she can maximize time with her kids in the morning before heading to work. "Breakfast is my favorite meal of the day, but it's the busiest time of day, too," she says. This simple morning meal can be topped with frozen fruit to keep things interesting regardless of what's in season.

ALMOND-BUTTER CHERRY-BERRY OVERNIGHT OATS

Serves 1

½ cup unsweetened vanilla almond milk

3 tablespoons creamy almond butter

1 tablespoon honey

2 ¼ teaspoons chia seeds

½ cup rolled oats

TOPPINGS

Frozen cherries, thawed

Frozen berries, thawed

Bee pollen (optional)

Other toppings of your choice

1. In a mason jar or small bowl, stir together the almond milk, almond butter, honey, chia seeds, and oats until thoroughly combined. Cover the mixture with a clean kitchen towel and refrigerate for at least 6 hours or up to overnight.

2. Uncover the mixture and top with the cherries, berries, bee pollen (if using), and any other toppings you desire. Enjoy.

Tip: If the almond butter thickens the oats too much overnight, add 2 tablespoons more almond milk to loosen them up in the morning.

DAIRY-FREE

LOW-INFLAMMATION

VEGETARIAN

BETTER DIGESTION

BETTER SLEEP

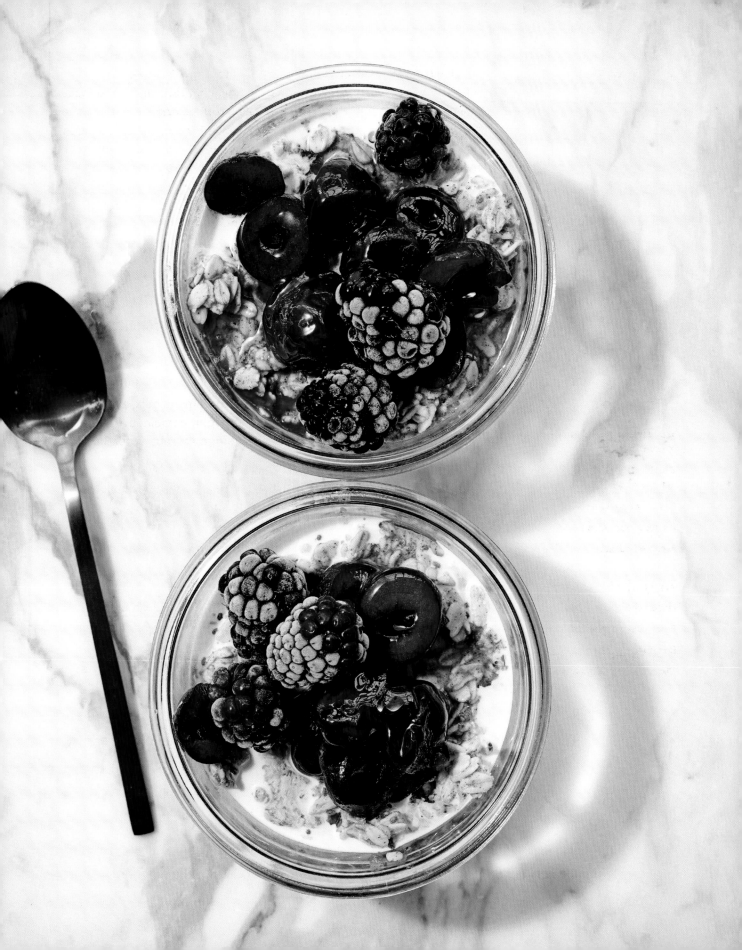

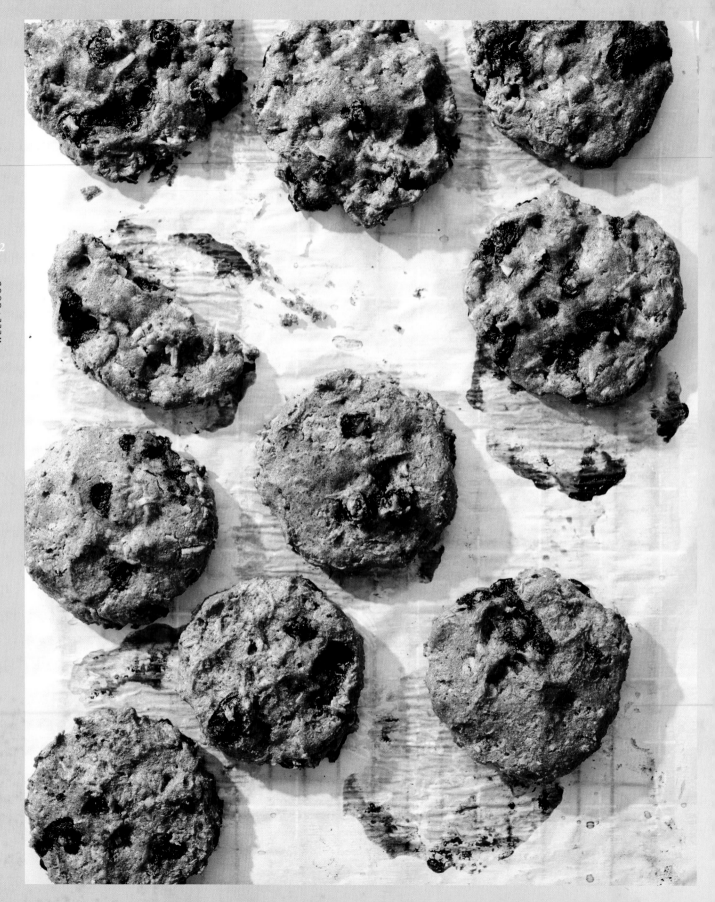

It can be difficult to eat a nourishing breakfast when busy mornings take over. "I love recipes like this that I can prep ahead of time," says Mark Hyman, MD, a mega-author, founder and medical director of the UltraWellness Center, and director of the Cleveland Clinic Center for Functional Medicine. "The healthy fats from coconut and almond butter with protein from pasture-raised eggs make these ultra-satiating, while the walnuts and blueberries provide powerful brain support to help me tackle my day." Don't let the word *cookie* fool you, though. There's no added sugar in these—they're naturally sweet thanks to real fruit, which also makes them super delish.

BLUEBERRY-FIG BREAKFAST COOKIES

Makes 12 to 14 cookies

¼ cup coconut flour

1 cup almond butter

3 tablespoons ground flaxseed

8 unsweetened, unsulphured dried figs, chopped

4 large eggs

2 tablespoons coconut milk, plus more if needed

1 tablespoon pure vanilla extract

1 tablespoon ground cinnamon

½ teaspoon sea salt

1 teaspoon baking soda

¾ cup unsweetened shredded coconut

1 cup fresh or thawed frozen blueberries

½ cup chopped raw walnuts

1. Preheat the oven to 350°F. Line a baking sheet with parchment paper.

2. In a food processor, combine the coconut flour, almond butter, flaxseed, figs, eggs, coconut milk, vanilla, cinnamon, salt, and baking soda. Process until all of the ingredients are well mixed and the figs are fully incorporated, adding more coconut milk as needed to reach the desired consistency.

3. Add the shredded coconut and pulse a few times just to incorporate it, but do not overprocess. Remove the blade and use a spatula to gently fold in the blueberries and walnuts.

4. Drop large spoonfuls of the dough onto the prepared baking sheet and spread them out flat with your fingers. (For a more uniform look, use an ice cream scoop, then press the balls of dough with the palm of your hand into flat, round cookies.)

5. Bake for 16 to 18 minutes, until golden brown. (Flatter cookies may take less time to bake, about 15 minutes.) Remove the pan from the oven. Let the cookies cool on the pan for 1 to 2 minutes, then transfer them to a wire rack to cool completely before serving or storing.

6. Cover the cookies with a clean kitchen towel overnight or store in an airtight container at room temperature for 3 to 4 days.

+

DAIRY-FREE

GLUTEN-FREE

LOW-INFLAMMATION

PALEO

VEGETARIAN

BETTER FOCUS

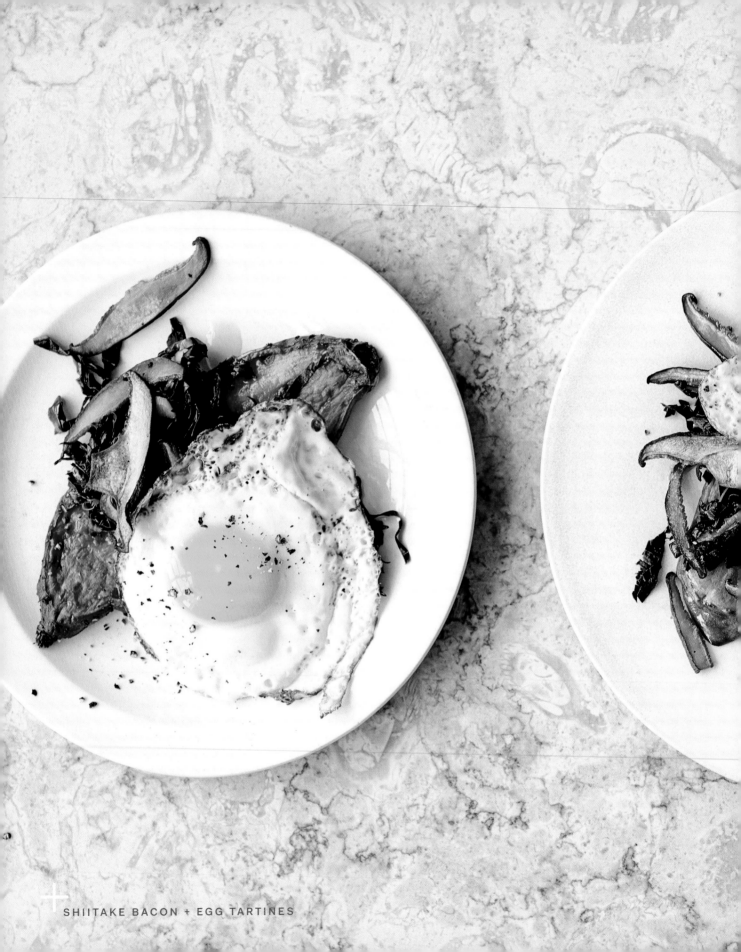

SHIITAKE BACON + EGG TARTINES

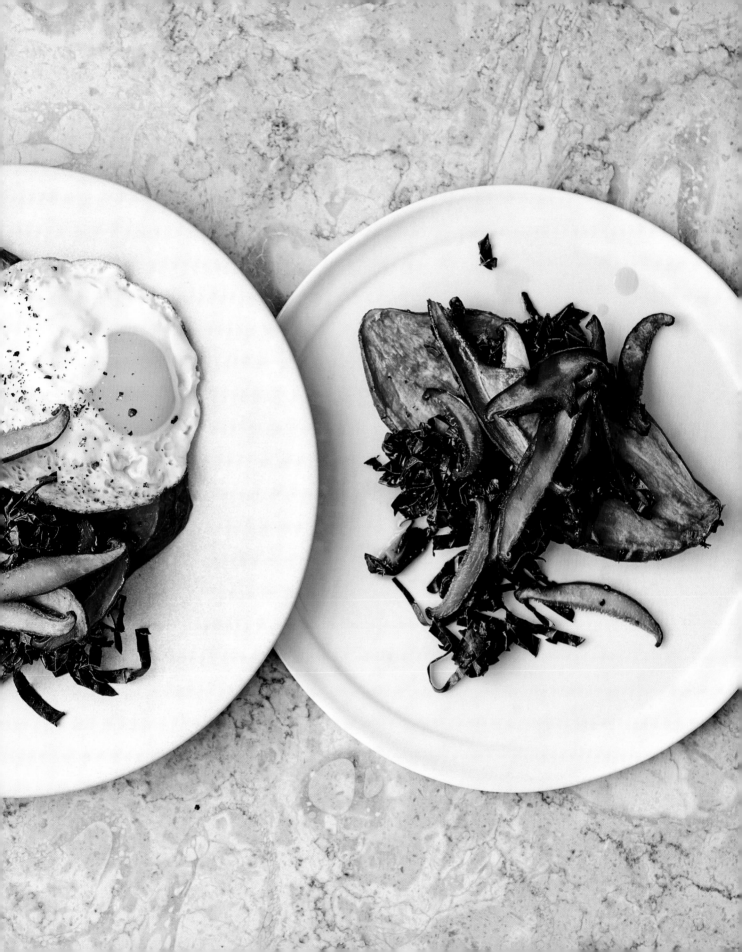

Lily Kunin, the super-popular *Clean Food Dirty City* blogger (who's the founder of Clean Market in New York and the author of *Good Clean Food*), is a pro at getting a nutrient-dense start to the day—*and* giving yourself room to improvise. "It's all about tuning into what foods make you feel healthy and vibrant," Lily says. Get creative with tartine toppings like avocado, "everything bagel" spice, raw sauerkraut, hot sauce, and whatever else makes you feel like taking on the world. Note: The sweet potato toasts keep well in the fridge, which comes in handy when you're trying to get out the door faster in the morning.

SHIITAKE BACON + EGG TARTINES

Makes 4 tartines

1 large sweet potato (preferably roundish), sliced lengthwise into planks about ½ inch thick

5 tablespoons extra-virgin olive oil

Pink Himalayan salt and freshly ground black pepper

10 shiitake mushrooms, or 1 (5-ounce) package, cleaned, stems trimmed, and thinly sliced

2 garlic cloves, thinly sliced

1 bunch Tuscan (lacinato or dinosaur) kale, stemmed, leaves thinly sliced

4 large eggs

½ teaspoon crushed red pepper flakes (optional)

DAIRY-FREE

GLUTEN-FREE

LOW-INFLAMMATION

PALEO

VEGETARIAN

BETTER MOOD

1. Preheat the oven to 375°F. Line two baking sheets with aluminum foil.

2. Arrange the sweet potato slices on one prepared baking sheet and drizzle ½ teaspoon of the olive oil on each side of each plank, and season with salt and black pepper. Roast for 35 minutes, flipping the sweet potatoes halfway through, until cooked through and golden. Remove the pan from the oven and let the sweet potatoes cool slightly before removing them from the pan.

3. Meanwhile, in a small bowl, toss the shiitakes with 1 tablespoon of the oil and a few generous pinches of salt and black pepper. Arrange them in an even layer on the other prepared baking sheet and bake for 15 to 20 minutes, until crispy.

4. Heat 2 tablespoons of the oil in a medium skillet over medium heat. When it shimmers, add the garlic and cook, stirring, for 1 minute, or until it begins to turn golden. Add the kale and cook, tossing, until just wilted, about 2 minutes. Season with salt and black pepper. Transfer the mixture to a bowl and cover with a clean kitchen towel to keep warm.

5. In the same skillet, heat the remaining oil over medium heat. When it shimmers, crack in 2 of the eggs, taking care to leave the yolks whole. Cook until the whites are just set, about 3 minutes, then turn off the heat and cover. Let sit until the whites are cooked through but the yolks are still runny, 1 to 2 minutes more. Remove from the heat and keep warm. Repeat with the remaining eggs.

6. Assemble the tartines. Divide the kale and shiitake bacon evenly among the sweet potato toasts and top each with one fried egg. Season the eggs with salt, black pepper, and red pepper flakes, if desired. Enjoy.

Dana James, MS, CNS, CDN, has a dream. The FoodCoach founder (who's a functional medicine nutritionist with a side of cognitive behavioral therapy training) and author of *The Archetype Diet* aims for the modern woman to be "free from the tyranny of diet dogma and self-doubt," starting with our relationship to food. "I want to live in a world where we instinctively know how to rebalance ourselves with food, nutrients, elixirs, mantras, and movement," she says. And every day is a new chance to move closer to that dream, so starting off her morning right is key. For Dana, that usually means protein—and this perfect and simple dish.

EASY HERB OMELET

Makes 1 omelet

3 large eggs

¼ teaspoon sea salt

¼ teaspoon freshly ground black pepper

2 ½ tablespoons finely chopped mixed fresh herbs, such as basil, dill, and parsley

1 teaspoon coconut oil

1. Crack the eggs into a small bowl and add the salt, pepper, 2 tablespoons of the herbs, and 1 tablespoon cold water. Gently whisk with a fork until the ingredients are fully incorporated and the mixture is slightly bubbly.

2. Melt the coconut oil in a small nonstick skillet over medium heat. When it shimmers, add the egg mixture. Cook, without moving, for about 1 minute, until the edges set and become white, then use a spatula to push them toward the center, tilting the pan to allow the uncooked egg to swirl into its place. Gently push and tilt the egg until the top of the omelet is mostly set, then use the spatula to fold the omelet in half to form a long cylinder shape.

3. Remove the omelet from heat and let sit for a few seconds, then transfer to a plate. Sprinkle the remaining herbs over the top and serve.

+

DAIRY-FREE

GLUTEN-FREE

KETOGENIC

LOW-FODMAP

LOW-INFLAMMATION

PALEO

VEGETARIAN

BETTER FOCUS

This recipe is what a lazy meal looks like to Jodi Moreno, the cookbook author, natural foods chef, and writer behind the acclaimed *What's Cooking Good Looking* blog. "There is an undeniable connection between health, beauty, well-being, and the food that we eat," she says. "Ingredients not only taste best when they are in their purest form, but they are also the best for you." True story: Jodi has been known to eat some of this egg bake for lunch, most of it for dinner, and finish it off the next day with a spoonful of chimichurri. Easy and delicious!

WHITE BEAN EGG BAKE

Serves 2 to 4

4 tablespoons extra-virgin olive oil

2 large handfuls of Swiss chard or spinach (about 3 ounces)

1 (15-ounce) can cannellini beans, drained and rinsed (or see Tip)

1 pint cherry tomatoes, halved

1 teaspoon paprika

½ teaspoon sea salt

1 teaspoon ground sumac (optional)

Freshly ground black pepper

4 large eggs

TOPPINGS

¼ cup mixed chopped fresh herbs, such as parsley, basil, or cilantro

1 or 2 scallions, sliced

¼ cup almonds, toasted (optional)

Tip: You can substitute 1½ cups cooked beans, if you prefer using dried (start with ½ cup dried beans to get about 1½ cups cooked). Chickpeas or black beans also taste just as delicious in the bake.

1. Place a medium cast-iron skillet in a cold oven and preheat the oven to 425°F.

2. In a large bowl, combine 3 tablespoons of the olive oil, the chard, beans, tomatoes, paprika, salt, sumac (if using), and pepper to taste. Toss to combine.

3. Remove the hot skillet from the oven and add the bean mixture. Shake to evenly distribute the mixture in the pan. Bake for about 15 minutes, until the chard has wilted and the tomatoes and beans are bubbling.

4. Transfer the skillet to the stovetop over medium-low heat. Using a spoon, make four wells in the mixture, then carefully break an egg into each. Cover the pan and cook for 5 to 10 minutes, until the egg whites are set but the yolks are still a bit runny.

5. Remove the skillet from the heat, top the bake with the herbs, scallions, and almonds, if desired. Serve immediately, or let cool completely, then transfer to a glass container and store in the refrigerator for 1 to 2 days.

DAIRY-FREE

GLUTEN-FREE

LOW-INFLAMMATION

VEGETARIAN

BETTER SKIN

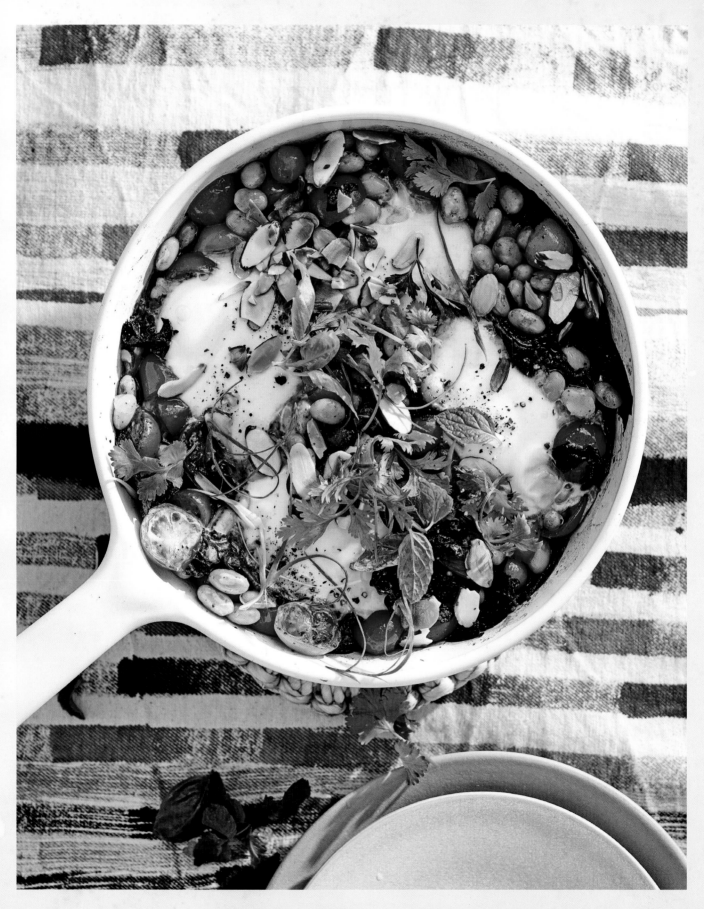

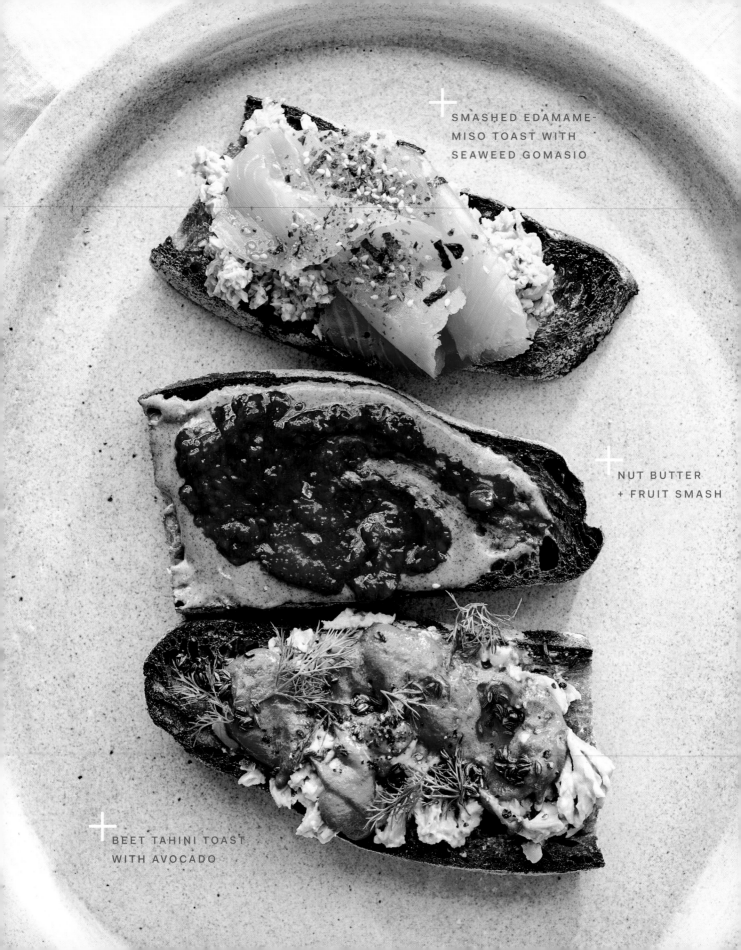

SMASHED EDAMAME-
MISO TOAST WITH
SEAWEED GOMASIO

NUT BUTTER
+ FRUIT SMASH

BEET TAHINI TOAST
WITH AVOCADO

ALISON CAYNE

Alison Cayne opened Haven's Kitchen (confession: It's a go-to of the Well+Good team)—a recreational cooking school and private event space in New York City—to give people the confidence that comes with being able to feed themselves well. "It's super empowering," says the cookbook author. "I also don't believe in categorizing foods—there are days for a *kitchari* cleanse and other days where nothing will beat a gooey chocolate cake." Alison created these three Insta-ready riffs to coax you out of your typical avocado toast routine—or at least upgrade your usual open-faced smash with a pretty beet tahini drizzle. Your followers (and your taste buds) will thank you.

BREAKFAST TOAST, THREE WAYS

SMASHED EDAMAME-MISO TOAST WITH SEAWEED GOMASIO

Makes about 4 toasts

Sea salt

1½ cups frozen shelled edamame

2 teaspoons white miso paste

Juice of 1 lime

1½ teaspoons toasted sesame oil

4 to 6 slices high-protein bread, toasted

4 ounces sliced smoked salmon (optional)

1 teaspoon seaweed gomasio

You can find seaweed *gomasio* (a sesame-salt mixture) online or in the spice aisle in grocery stores. This recipe makes 1½ cups edamame mixture.

1. Fill a small pot with 3 to 4 cups water and salt it well. Bring to a boil over high heat. Add the edamame and cook for 10 minutes, until you can smush them with your fingers. Drain, reserving the cooking liquid, and transfer the edamame to a medium bowl.

2. Add the miso, lime juice, sesame oil, and 2 teaspoons of the reserved edamame cooking liquid. Using a fork or a mortar and pestle, smash the edamame until the mixture is a spreadable paste.

3. Spread the mixture on the toast, top with the salmon, if desired, and the gomasio, and serve.

recipes continue

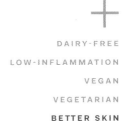

DAIRY-FREE

LOW-INFLAMMATION

VEGAN

VEGETARIAN

BETTER SKIN

NUT BUTTER
+ FRUIT SMASH

Alison takes a good thing (PB+J) and makes it BFY ("better for you") by creating her own compote from scratch. Frozen berries will take longer to come to a boil, but can be simmered in the same fashion as fresh, ultimately yielding 1⅓ cups fruit compote.

Makes 4 to 6 toasts

3 cups fresh or frozen mixed berries and/or cubed pitted stone fruit

1 tablespoon honey, plus more to taste

Juice of ½ lemon (about 1 tablespoon)

4 to 6 tablespoons nut butter of your choice

4 to 6 slices high-protein bread, toasted

Sea salt, for sprinkling

1. In a medium saucepan, combine the fruit, honey, and lemon juice. Bring to a boil over high heat, then reduce the heat to medium and simmer, stirring often, for 10 minutes, or until the mixture thickens and takes on a gooey, jammy texture. Remove the pan from the heat and let the compote cool for about 15 minutes.

2. Spread 1 tablespoon of the nut butter on each piece of toast, then drizzle with 1½ tablespoons of the compote and sprinkle with salt before serving.

3. Store leftover compote in an airtight container in the refrigerator for up to 1 week or in the freezer for up to 6 months.

DAIRY-FREE

LOW-INFLAMMATION

VEGETARIAN

BETTER ENERGY

BEET TAHINI TOAST WITH AVOCADO

"I consider this recipe a treat, not a daily must-have," Alison notes. This gorgeous green-and-red combo makes about 1¾ cups of beet tahini.

Makes 4 to 6 toasts

FOR THE BEET TAHINI

2 tablespoons red wine vinegar

1 large beet, scrubbed

2 tablespoons olive oil, plus more as needed

¼ teaspoon sea salt, plus more as needed

¼ cup tahini

Juice of 1 lemon (2 to 4 tablespoons)

FOR THE TOASTS

2 small avocados, pitted and peeled

4 to 6 slices high-protein bread, toasted

1 lemon wedge

Sea salt

1 teaspoon cumin seeds (optional)

Olive oil, for drizzling (optional)

1. Make the beet tahini. Preheat the oven to 400°F.

2. Pour the vinegar and ½ cup water onto a rimmed baking sheet. Rub the beet with olive oil and season with a pinch of salt, then tightly wrap it in aluminum foil and place it on the baking sheet. Roast for 1 hour, or until the beet is cooked all the way through and can be easily pierced with a knife. Let the beet sit until cool enough to handle, but while it's still warm, use your thumbs to rub off the skin.

3. Coarsely chop the skinless beet and transfer to a blender or food processor. Add the tahini, lemon juice, olive oil, salt, and 3 tablespoons water. Blend until the mixture is smooth and easy to drizzle, adding more water, 1½ teaspoons water at a time, as needed to reach the desired consistency.

4. Assemble the toasts. In a small bowl, use a fork to smash the avocado, then spread a bit onto each piece of toast. Squeeze over a bit of lemon juice and add a pinch of salt. Drizzle the beet tahini on top. Sprinkle with the cumin seeds and drizzle with olive oil, if desired. Enjoy or refrigerate leftover beet tahini for up to 5 days.

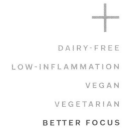

DAIRY-FREE

LOW-INFLAMMATION

VEGAN

VEGETARIAN

BETTER FOCUS

This blender recipe was born when the healing principles Federica Norreri learned in Ayurvedic Nutrition and Culinary Training met the reality of her busy lifestyle. So she Ayurveda-ized what we traditionally think of as waffles— you know, full of flour, absent of nutrients, and topped with sugar-loaded syrup—to become more nourishing and more easily digestible. "The idea that you can make any recipe, from any cuisine, have healing benefits, is one I live by each and every day," says the Italian-born-and-raised cook. This breakfast revamp was so genius, it's now on the menu at Divya's Kitchen, an Ayurveda-inspired, largely gluten-free eatery in New York.

SAVORY RED LENTIL WAFFLES

Makes 4 waffles

FOR THE WAFFLES

½ cup red lentils

⅓ cup rice flour, plus more as needed

2 tablespoons amaranth flour

2 tablespoons arrowroot powder

1 teaspoon baking powder

¼ teaspoon baking soda

¼ teaspoon sea salt

1 teaspoon ghee or coconut oil, plus more for greasing

¼ teaspoon ground turmeric

1 cup buttermilk or vegan yogurt

1 tablespoon fresh lime juice (from about ½ lime)

DAIRY-FREE

GLUTEN-FREE

LOW-INFLAMMATION

VEGAN

VEGETARIAN

BETTER FOCUS

FOR THE BLUEBERRY COMPOTE

1 cup fresh or frozen blueberries

1 tablespoon raw sugar

1 star anise pod, or ⅛ teaspoon ground star anise

Pure maple syrup, for serving

Vegan whipped cream, for serving

1. Make the waffles. Put the lentils in a medium bowl and add water to cover. Refrigerate overnight, then drain very well.

2. Heat a waffle maker to medium-high.

3. In a blender or a food processor, combine the lentils, rice flour, amaranth flour, arrowroot, baking powder, baking soda, and salt. (Don't blend yet.)

4. Melt the ghee in a small cast-iron skillet over medium-low heat. Add the turmeric and cook for 3 or 4 seconds, until it reaches a deep golden color. Transfer the spiced ghee to a medium bowl and whisk in the buttermilk or vegan yogurt and lime juice.

5. Add the buttermilk mixture to the blender and blend until completely smooth. If the mixture is too thick, add water or more buttermilk as needed; if it's too thin, add 1 tablespoon rice flour.

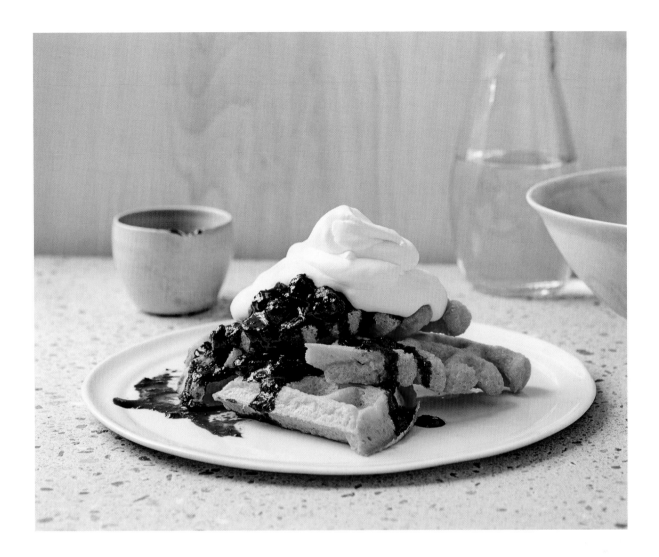

6. When the waffle maker is heated, grease its plates with ghee and pour in one-quarter of the batter. Close the waffle maker and cook until golden brown. Transfer the waffle to a plate and repeat with the remaining batter to make 4 waffles total.

7. Meanwhile, make the blueberry compote. In a small pot, combine the blueberries, sugar, and star anise and cook over medium-low heat for about 5 minutes, or until the blueberries break down a bit and reach a jam-like consistency. Remove the pot from the heat and set aside. If you used a whole star anise, discard it.

8. Serve the waffles with the blueberry compote, maple syrup, and whipped cream alongside.

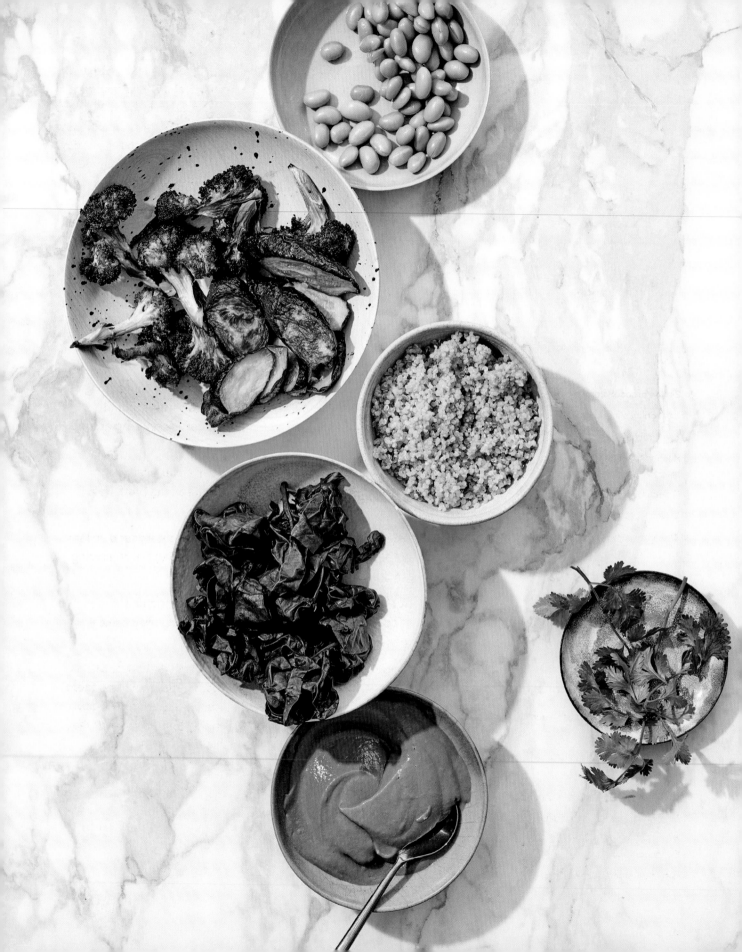

MADELEINE
MURPHY

Lean, clean, and green is how Madeleine Murphy—cofounder of Montauk Juice Factory and The End Brooklyn (whose whimsical unicorn-inspired creations put it on the map)—describes this super-satisfying meal. "I love to double this recipe so I have extra for another quick breakfast or lunch," says the certified holistic health coach. If you make this, "you will start your day nourished, energized, light, and glowing—the way every goddess should!" As a fan of functional foods that support women, Maddie created the hormone-balancing green sauce (avocado and flax for the win), over a base of fiber, veggies, and healthy fats.

GREEN GODDESS BREAKFAST BOWL

Serves 2

2 cups broccoli florets

1 zucchini, sliced

3 to 4 tablespoons olive oil

Kosher salt and freshly ground black pepper

½ cup uncooked quinoa

1 cup vegetable broth

2 cups chopped Swiss chard leaves

FOR THE SAUCE

1 avocado, pitted and peeled

1 cup packed mixed fresh parsley and basil leaves

2 garlic cloves

¼ cup olive oil

¼ cup flaxseed oil

2 tablespoons fresh lemon juice

1 teaspoon sea salt

TO ASSEMBLE

½ cup shelled edamame, steamed

1 avocado, pitted, peeled, sliced

4 large eggs, cooked to your liking (optional)

¼ cup chopped fresh cilantro

1. Preheat the oven to 450°F.

2. Arrange the broccoli florets and sliced zucchini on a rimmed baking sheet and drizzle with the olive oil. Season generously with salt and pepper. Roast for 15 to 20 minutes, until the broccoli is browning around the edges and the zucchini is crispy.

3. In a medium pot, combine the quinoa and broth, cover, and cook over medium-low heat for about 20 minutes, or until all the broth has been absorbed.

4. Meanwhile, place the chard in a large pot. Add ¼ cup water and season liberally with salt and pepper. Cover and cook over medium heat, stirring occasionally, until the chard has wilted, about 4 minutes.

5. Make the green goddess sauce. In a food processor or blender, combine the avocado, herbs, garlic, olive oil, flaxseed oil, lemon juice, and salt. Process until smooth.

6. Assemble the bowls. Divide the quinoa between two shallow bowls. Add the roasted broccoli, zucchini, chard, and edamame, arranging them in separate piles. Fan the avocado slices over the veggies. Top each bowl with 2 cooked eggs, if desired. Spoon the green goddess sauce over the top and garnish with the cilantro before serving.

7. Store any leftover sauce refrigerated in an airtight container for up to 1 week.

+

DAIRY-FREE

GLUTEN-FREE

VEGAN

VEGETARIAN

BETTER DIGESTION

BETTER SEX

Summer Rayne Oakes, known as a garden goddess (thanks to the glorious urban oasis she documents on her YouTube channel, Homestead Brooklyn) is also a professional sweet tooth problem-solver. "I had always been saddled with one, so I began discovering how to eat better by changing my approach," says the certified holistic nutritionist and founder of SugarDetoxMe (and author of the book of the same title). "This recipe is like a snack, breakfast, and dessert in one. It's light and full of flavor—and the sweetness of the grapefruit is brought out through broiling." The cook time will depend on your oven, so keep an eye on the edges as they heat.

BROILED GINGER-CINNAMON GRAPEFRUIT

Serves 2

½ teaspoon pureed fresh ginger

½ teaspoon ground cinnamon

Sea salt

1 large grapefruit, halved crosswise

2 teaspoons raw pistachios, crushed

4 tablespoons vegan coconut yogurt

4 fresh mint leaves, finely chopped

1. Preheat the broiler with a rack positioned 4 inches from the heat source.

2. Using your fingers or a pastry brush, spread ¼ teaspoon of the ginger, ¼ teaspoon of the cinnamon, and a pinch of salt over the cut side of each grapefruit half. Place the halves cut-side up on a baking sheet or in a baking dish.

3. Broil the grapefruit for about 3 minutes, or until the edges of the peel begin to brown.

4. Remove from the oven and top with the pistachios, yogurt, and mint leaves, dividing them evenly. Serve warm.

DAIRY-FREE

GLUTEN-FREE

PALEO

VEGAN

VEGETARIAN

BETTER SEX

BETTER SKIN

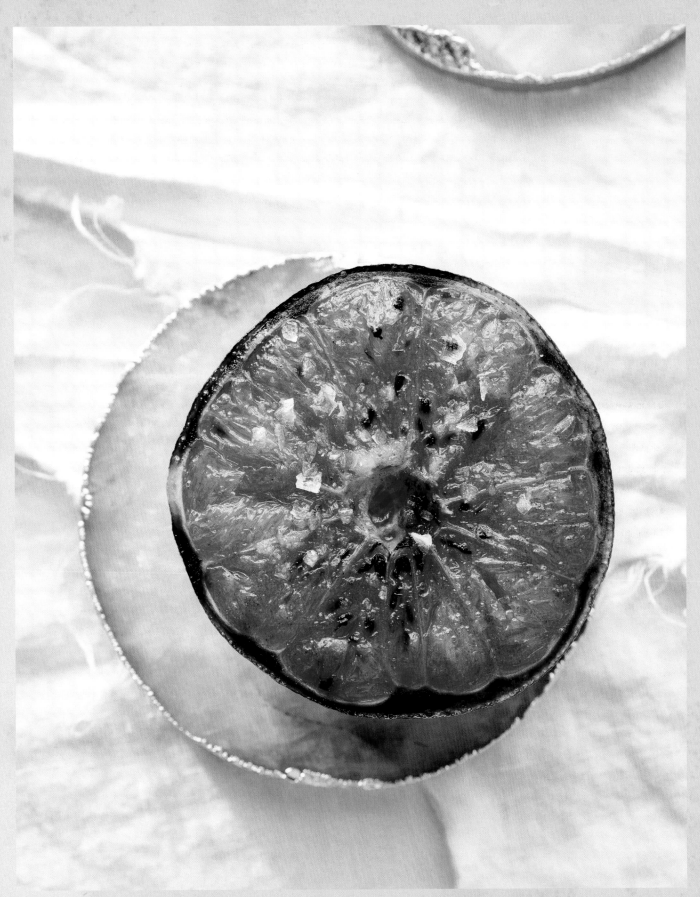

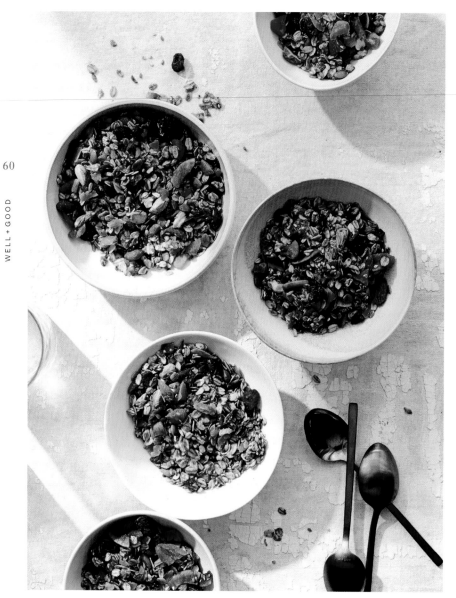

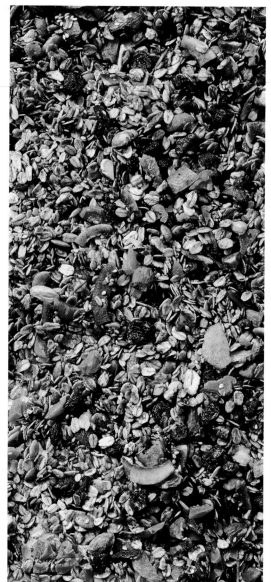

The second this granola hits the oven, you'll understand how it earned its name. Celebrity wellness maven, doula, and Well+Good Council member Latham Thomas choreographed this glow-inducing recipe to take center stage right away, with enough leftovers to last until you're ready to treat yourself to the next batch. "What we eat becomes our blood, our thoughts, and our actions," says the founder of Mama Glow, a lifestyle brand, book, and website for holistic expectant and new moms. Her mantra: "Be kind to yourself and be mindful about what you choose to eat."

ROCK + ROLL GRANOLA

Makes about 7 cups

¼ cup packed light brown sugar

¼ cup grapeseed oil

2 tablespoons honey

1 tablespoon pure maple syrup

2 teaspoons pure vanilla extract

2 teaspoons ground cinnamon

1 teaspoon sea salt

½ cup mixed nuts, such as pistachios and almonds, toasted and coarsely chopped

3 tablespoons flaxseed

3 tablespoons sesame seeds

¼ cup raw sunflower or pumpkin seeds

½ cup unsweetened coconut flakes

3½ cups rolled oats

2 cups chopped mixed dried fruit, such as dried cherries and cranberries

1. Preheat the oven to 375°F. Line a rimmed baking sheet with aluminum foil.

2. In a large bowl, combine the brown sugar, grapeseed oil, honey, maple syrup, vanilla, cinnamon, and salt. Stir to fully incorporate, then fold in the mixed nuts, flaxseed, sesame seeds, sunflower seeds, coconut flakes, and oats. Stir well to fully coat the solid ingredients.

3. Spread the mixture into an even layer over the prepared baking sheet. Bake for 10 minutes, then stir. Bake for 10 to 15 minutes more, until the granola is golden brown and toasted to your liking.

4. Remove from the oven and let the granola cool on the pan for 10 minutes, then stir in the dried fruit. Let cool for 5 to 10 minutes more and enjoy warm, or let cool completely before storing in an airtight container in a cool, dry spot for up to 2 months.

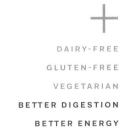

DAIRY-FREE

GLUTEN-FREE

VEGETARIAN

BETTER DIGESTION

BETTER ENERGY

Farmer-foodie Andrea Bemis had a hard time naming this baked cauliflower concoction. "Sounds weird, I know, but trust me, these little 'bagels' are awesome!" says the *Dishing Up the Dirt* blogger (and author of a cookbook of the same name). She loves to slice them in half and spread mashed avocado on each side. Try that, or keep it simple with a smear of grass-fed butter for a Paleo-friendly breakfast. Either way, we recommend you eat them fresh from the oven like Andrea does at her Tumbleweed Farm home in Oregon.

ZA'ATAR-SPICED CAULIFLOWER BAGELS

Makes 6 bagels

1 medium head cauliflower, broken into florets (3 to 4 cups; or see Tip)

2 tablespoons almond flour

2 tablespoons coconut flour

¼ teaspoon garlic powder

1 teaspoon kosher salt

2 large eggs, lightly beaten

Za'atar seasoning, for sprinkling

1. Preheat the oven to 400°F. Line a baking sheet with parchment paper.

2. In a food processor, pulse the cauliflower florets until broken down to a fine, rice-like consistency.

3. In a medium bowl, combine the almond flour, coconut flour, garlic powder, salt, and eggs. Stir in the riced cauliflower and mix until thoroughly combined.

4. Using your hands, form the dough into about six 3-inch rounds and place them on the prepared baking sheet. Use your finger to poke a hole in the centers, like a traditional bagel. Sprinkle with za'atar and bake for 30 minutes, or until golden brown around the edges.

5. Serve the bagels warm, or transfer to a resealable plastic bag and store in the refrigerator for up to 3 days or in the freezer for up to 1 month.

Tip: Use 3 to 4 cups prepared cauliflower rice (available in the produce or freezer section at your grocery store) for quicker prep.

DAIRY-FREE

GLUTEN-FREE

LOW-INFLAMMATION

PALEO

VEGETARIAN

BETTER FOCUS

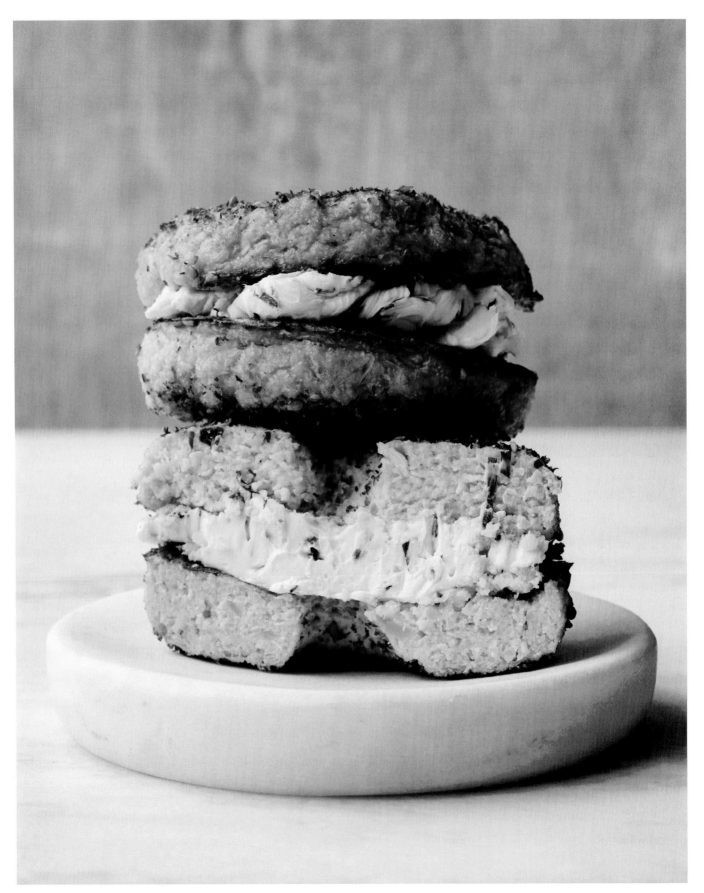

SMOOTHIES + SMOOTHIE BOWLS

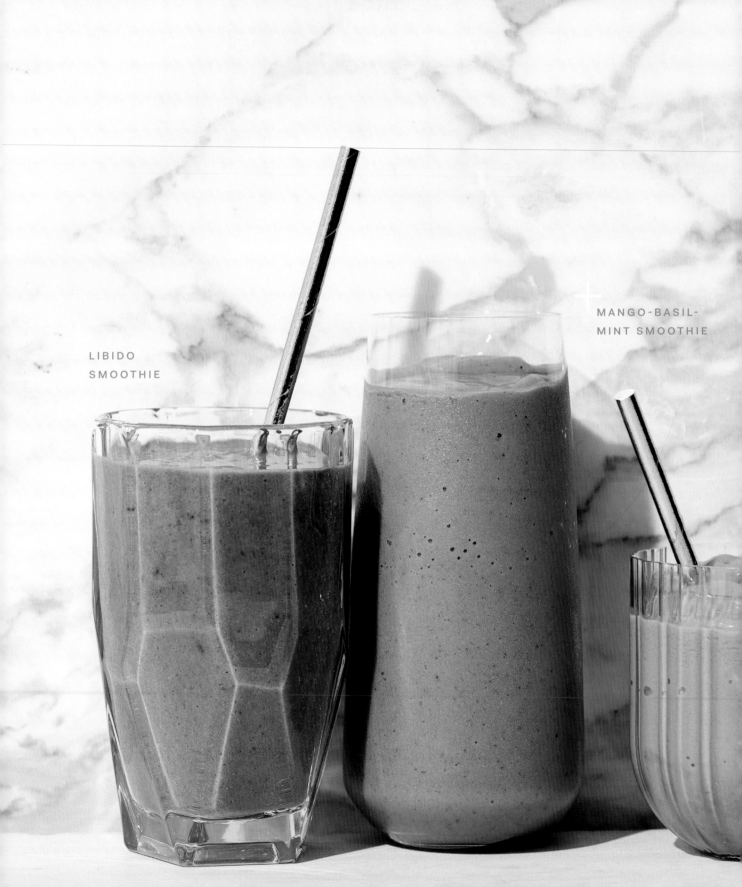

LIBIDO
SMOOTHIE

MANGO-BASIL-
MINT SMOOTHIE

LILA
DARVILLE

"As a sex and intimacy coach, my work is about bringing the body into a state of vitality—both in and out of bed," says Well+Good Council member Lila Darville, who created this smoothie to help balance the hormone cycles that support a vital sex life. The busy mom's hassle-free tonic for the sexually empowered is as easy as blending greens, berries, and cacao—and yes, it's as chocolaty and delicious as it sounds. "Eating should be healthy, but it should also be a pleasure," says Lila. "There is a direct correlation between the amount of pleasure you experience in life and the amount you experience in sex." We'll get out the blender right now.

LIBIDO SMOOTHIE

Serves 1

1 cup baby kale or spinach

2 cups nondairy milk or water

½ cup frozen blackberries

1 tablespoon raw cacao powder

½ frozen banana

1 teaspoon mushroom blend powder

1 teaspoon maca powder

Local raw honey or dates, such as Medjool or Deglet Noor

1 teaspoon schisandra berries (optional; see Tip)

1. In a high-speed blender, combine the kale, nondairy milk, blackberries, cacao powder, banana, mushroom blend powder, maca, honey or dates, and schisandra. Blend until completely smooth.

2. Pour the smoothie into a glass and enjoy immediately.

Tip: Find schisandra berries (often called magnolia berries or five-flavor fruit) online or in Chinese herbal shops.

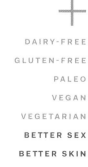

DAIRY-FREE

GLUTEN-FREE

PALEO

VEGAN

VEGETARIAN

BETTER SEX

BETTER SKIN

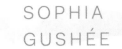
Healthy home guru Sophia Gushée is all about making over living spaces to create toxin-free sanctuaries (or, at least, as close to toxin-free as you can get). But when she wants to create a happy home—as in, her own—she reaches for this concoction. "My kids think they're eating peppermint ice cream," says the Well+Good Council member, author, and founder of Ruan Living. She serves this as a breakfast or as an afternoon snack, jamming in as many nutrients as she can get away with. You can adjust the spinach and basil to taste for sensitive eaters, though the natural sweetness of the mango and oomph of the essential oil hide almost everything else.

MANGO-BASIL-MINT SMOOTHIE

Serves 1

3 cups chopped frozen mango

½ cup fresh basil leaves

2 large handfuls of spinach

1 tablespoon raw honey

1 or 2 drops food-grade peppermint essential oil

½ cup unsweetened coconut water or non-dairy milk, plus more as needed (see Tip)

Fresh lime juice (optional)

1. In a high-speed blender, combine the mango, basil, spinach, honey, peppermint oil, coconut water, and lime juice (if using). Blend until completely smooth, adding more liquid as needed (see Tip), until the desired consistency is reached.

2. Pour into a glass and enjoy, or transfer to an airtight container and freeze for up to 3 months.

Tip: If you need more liquid to help blend your smoothie, a small amount of cold-pressed green juice or kefir is a nice addition.

DAIRY-FREE

GLUTEN-FREE

LOW-INFLAMMATION

PALEO

VEGETARIAN

BETTER SKIN

When Lianna Sugarman made her first green smoothie, a total life overhaul followed. "That day created a seismic shift in my relationship with food, cravings, and my body—and one that totally changed my career forever," says the founder of LuliTonix, which offers blended—not pressed—evolved juices and "other cool and magical shit." This total wellness recipe uses olive oil and a bit of salt, which—when combined with creamy avocado, the earthiness of greens, acid from the lemon, and the subtle sweetness of the fennel— makes for a zero-grams-of-sugar foodie-friendly blend. "It keeps me satiated, energized, and glowy through my afternoon slump," Lianna says.

TUSCAN GLOW SMOOTHIE

Serves 1

1 cup packed spinach

¼ cup chopped or sliced fennel

¼ medium avocado, pitted and peeled

1 (1-inch) strip lemon zest (peeled with a vegetable peeler), washed

Juice of ½ large lemon (1 to 1½ tablespoons)

⅛ teaspoon pink Himalayan salt

1 tablespoon extra-virgin olive oil

¼ cup ice cubes (see Tip)

1. In a high-speed blender, combine the spinach, fennel, avocado, lemon zest, lemon juice, salt, olive oil, ice (if using), and ¼ cup water. Blend well, moving from low to high speed and using the tamper as needed, until smooth. Add more water as needed to reach the desired consistency.

2. Pour into a glass and enjoy.

Tip: If you want to prep the recipe an hour or so ahead of time, say, before you head out to work, blend in the ice just before drinking the smoothie.

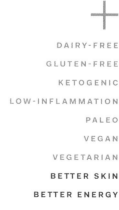

DAIRY-FREE

GLUTEN-FREE

KETOGENIC

LOW-INFLAMMATION

PALEO

VEGAN

VEGETARIAN

BETTER SKIN

BETTER ENERGY

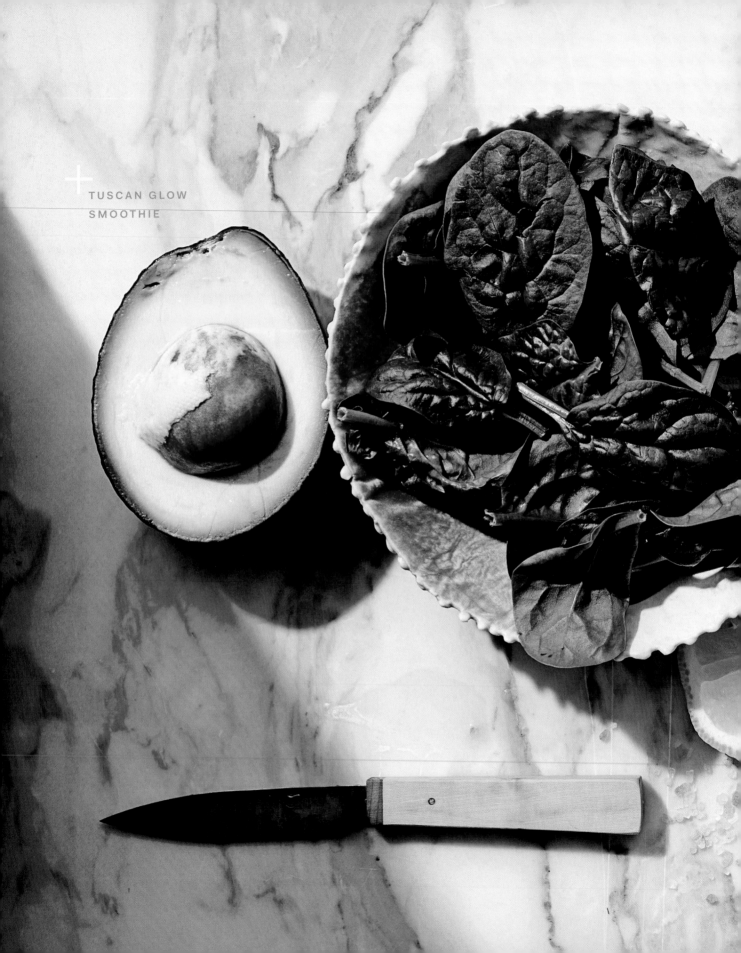

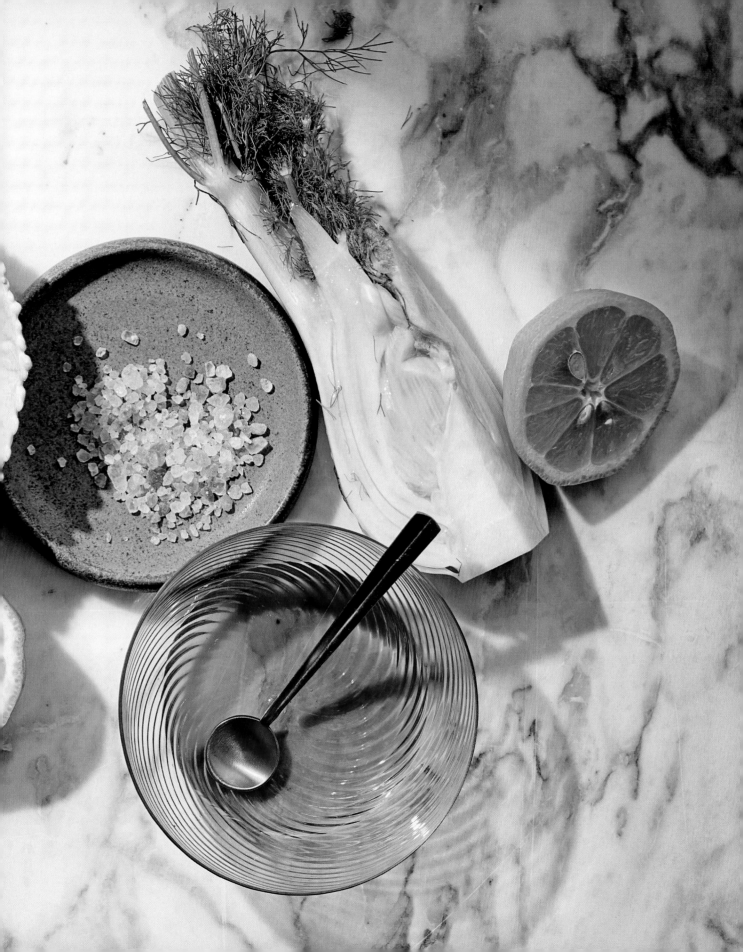

When fitness phenom Kayla Itsines leaves the house, she tends to cause a scene—her in-person boot camp class has been known to draw thousands of fans. Kayla feels her best when she gets a good start at home, making her own meals using healthy foods rich in nutrients. "It is really important for me to fuel my body properly," says the co-creator of the Bikini Body Guide and the SWEAT training app. Waking up with this colorful bowl means Kayla eats a range of different foods to give her the energy she needs to tackle any high-intensity BBG workout and feel great. "And it's super pretty," she adds.

RASPBERRY-PEACH SMOOTHIE BOWL

Serves 1

1 frozen banana, sliced

½ cup frozen strawberries

½ medium peach, pitted

½ cup low-fat plain yogurt (see Tip)

⅓ cup low-fat milk or nondairy milk

½ teaspoon pure vanilla extract

TOPPINGS

1 tablespoon slivered almonds, toasted

1 tablespoon unsweetened coconut flakes, toasted

½ medium peach, pitted and thinly sliced

6 to 8 fresh raspberries

1 teaspoon chia seeds

1. In a high-speed blender, combine the banana, strawberries, peach, yogurt, milk, and vanilla. Blend until completely smooth.

2. Pour the smoothie mixture into a bowl and top with the toasted almonds, coconut flakes, peach slices, raspberries, and chia seeds.

Tip: Swap in almond or cashew yogurt for a nondairy, vegan option.

DAIRY-FREE

GLUTEN-FREE

LOW-INFLAMMATION

PALEO

VEGAN

VEGETARIAN

BETTER MOOD

BETTER SKIN

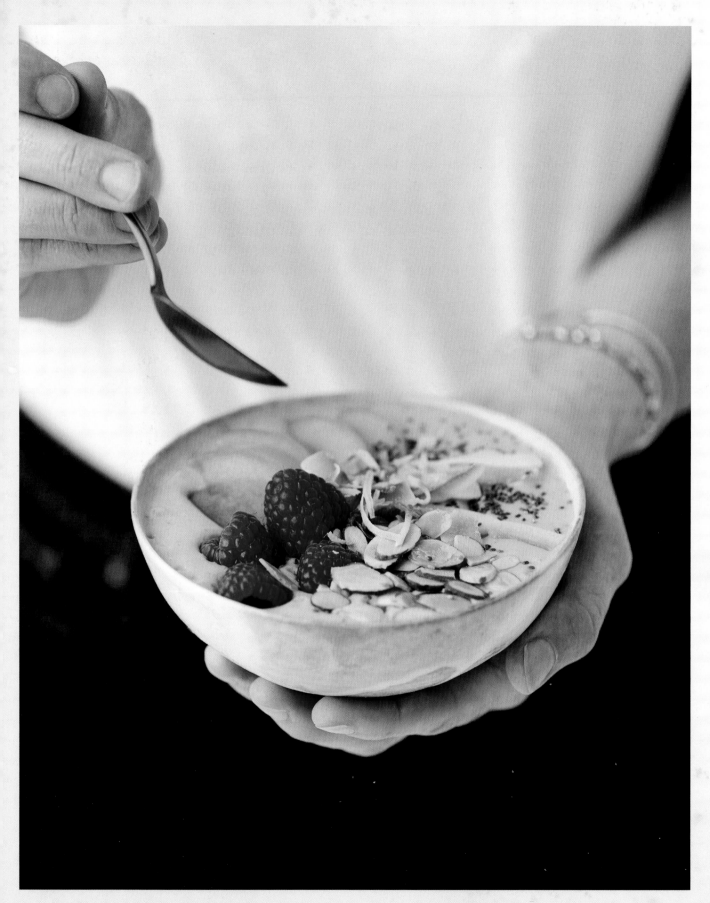

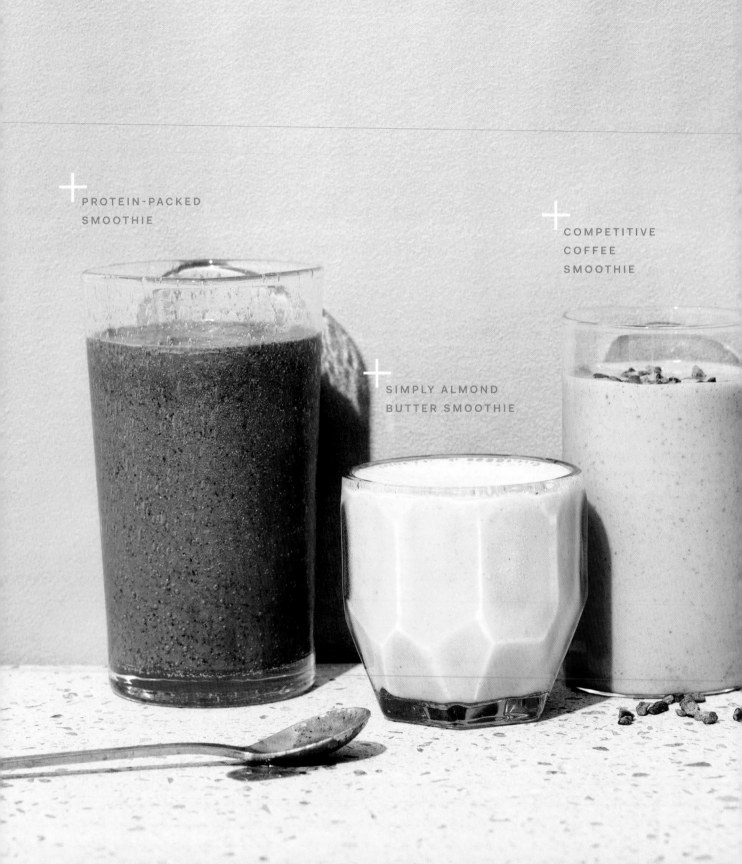

+ PROTEIN-PACKED
  SMOOTHIE

+ COMPETITIVE
  COFFEE
  SMOOTHIE

+ SIMPLY ALMOND
  BUTTER SMOOTHIE

Well+Good Council member Robin Berzin, MD, likes to eat in a style that she calls plant-based Paleo. As the founder and CEO of Parsley Health, a medical practice with a whole-body approach, she focuses on getting protein, greens, and a healthy fat at every meal, and generally avoids dairy, gluten, soy, excess alcohol, and processed foods. "This diet leaves me energized, balances my hormones, and keeps inflammation low," she says. Dr. Berzin suggests drinking this specific blend whenever you feel a sugar craving coming on, but it's also basic enough for customizing with what your body needs in the moment, like extra leafy greens or added protein.

PROTEIN-PACKED SMOOTHIE

Serves 1

1 to 2 tablespoons sugar-free protein powder

½ cup nondairy milk

⅓ cup frozen blueberries

⅓ cup frozen raspberries

1 tablespoon almond butter

1 cup spinach

Ice, as desired

1. In a high-speed blender, combine the protein powder, nondairy milk, blueberries, raspberries, almond butter, spinach, and ice (if using). Blend until smooth and completely combined, adding water as needed to reach the desired consistency.

2. Pour into a glass and enjoy.

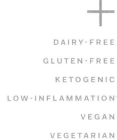

DAIRY-FREE

GLUTEN-FREE

KETOGENIC

LOW-INFLAMMATION

VEGAN

VEGETARIAN

BETTER ENERGY

BETTER FOCUS

For Barry's Bootcamp CEO Joey Gonzalez, keeping it simple at mealtime is a must. He's leading a growing fitness empire, first of all. And the Well+Good Council member still somehow teaches classes every week— all while balancing family time with his husband and kids in Los Angeles. "Choosing when to eat is as important as what to eat," he says. This recipe gives you a taste of the nut butter smoothie from the Fuel Bar inside Barry's, but to truly channel your inner Joey, swap out the whey protein for bone broth powder (though he warns that the taste isn't for everyone).

SIMPLY ALMOND BUTTER SMOOTHIE

Serves 1

1½ cups unsweetened almond milk, plus more as needed

1 cup sliced bananas

3 tablespoons almond butter

1 scoop vanilla whey protein or bone broth protein powder

1 cup ice cubes

1. In a high-speed blender, combine the almond milk, bananas, almond butter, vanilla whey, and ice. Blend until smooth, adding more almond milk as needed to reach your desired texture.

2. Pour into a glass and enjoy.

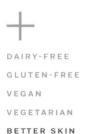

DAIRY-FREE

GLUTEN-FREE

VEGAN

VEGETARIAN

BETTER SKIN

While training as a competitive boxer, Marcus Antebi altered his diet to consist primarily of cold-pressed juices, smoothies, and salads. This lifestyle change (along with a dissatisfaction with his fueling options) led him to open the very first Juice Press location in 2010. (There are now 80 or so.) "Eliminating processed foods and replacing them with pure, plant-based options has given me the physical health to succeed as a Muay Thai boxer and yogi," he says. Marcus's smoothie recipe is an excellent pick-me-up for early-morning workouts, with coffee and cauliflower for serious mental clarity. It's plant power—with a punch.

COMPETITIVE COFFEE SMOOTHIE

Serves 1

¾ cup brewed coffee, cold

¼ cup nondairy milk

½ frozen banana

¼ cup chopped frozen cauliflower

¼ cup ice cubes

2 pitted dates, such as Medjool or Deglet Noor

2 tablespoons almond butter (optional)

Chopped cacao nibs and melted almond butter, for topping

1. In a high-speed blender, combine the coffee, nondairy milk, banana, cauliflower, ice, dates, and almond butter (if using). Blend until smooth, creamy, and completely combined.

2. Pour into a glass and top with cacao nibs and a drizzle of melted almond butter. Enjoy immediately.

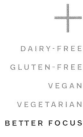

DAIRY-FREE

GLUTEN-FREE

VEGAN

VEGETARIAN

BETTER FOCUS

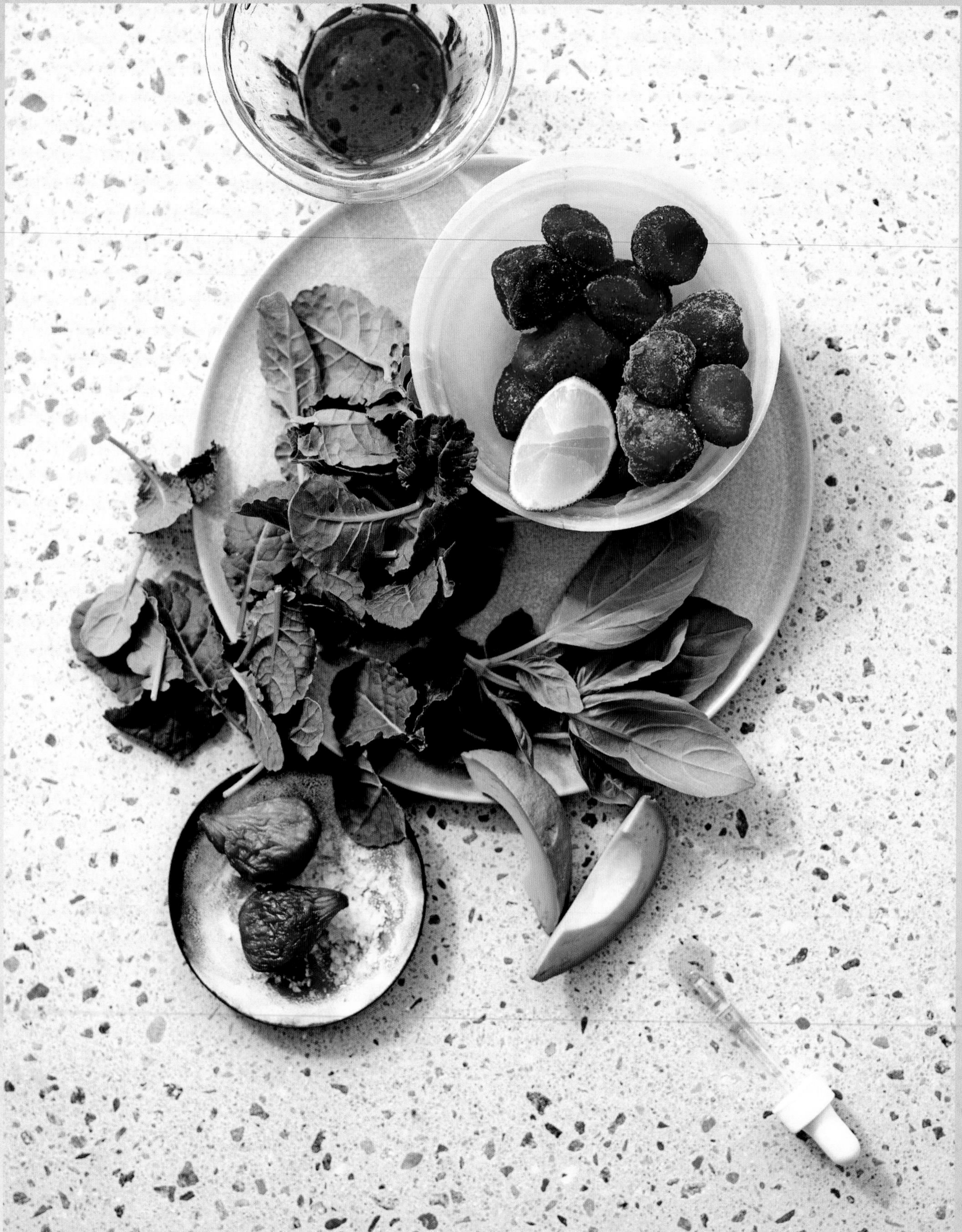

Well+Good cofounder Alexia Brue's smoothies went from gloppy, unbalanced purees to soufflé-like dream greens thanks to her spiritual-blends guide, Lianna Sugarman. "She taught me the right proportion of liquid to produce, so I always nail the texture now," says the wellness-media maven. Alexia calls this mixture her early-morning salad, which grounds her before a fitness or yoga class. The concoction includes a drop of CBD oil, which is said to relieve inflammation and decrease anxiety. You can also leave the tops on the fresh strawberries for an extra boost of greens.

STRAWBERRY CBD SMOOTHIE

Serves 1

1 cup packed kale leaves or other dark leafy green

¼ cup packed fresh basil leaves

⅓ cup fresh or frozen strawberries, tops included

¼ medium avocado, pitted and peeled

1 dried fig

Juice of ½ lime (about 1 tablespoon)

¼ teaspoon sea salt

1 tablespoon honey, pure maple syrup, or agave nectar (optional)

1 drop high-quality CBD oil (optional)

¼ cup ice cubes

1. In a high-speed blender, combine the kale, basil, strawberries, avocado, fig, lime juice, salt, honey (if using), CBD oil (if using), and ½ cup water. Blend until smooth.

2. Pour into a glass over ice and enjoy, or pour into a jar or bottle with a lid, store in the refrigerator, and drink within a couple of hours. Shake well before drinking.

+

DAIRY-FREE

GLUTEN-FREE

LOW-INFLAMMATION

PALEO

VEGAN

VEGETARIAN

BETTER MOOD

BETTER SKIN

EAT FOR BETTER MOOD

If you experience big mood swings, or you feel anxious or depressed on a regular basis, the way you eat can make a huge difference in changing the way you feel. I've seen it countless times in my experience with clients at the holistic FLO Living Hormone Center in New York City. And in my experience, our mood gets thrown off for three reasons:

HORMONES. For women, when estrogen and progesterone are out of balance, it can wreak havoc on your mood. Addressing underlying issues can improve your emotional well-being— and one of the most effective ways to address hormone imbalances is with food.

So what causes hormone imbalances? A big factor is imbalanced blood sugar. This can happen if you skip meals, don't eat enough healthy fat, don't eat enough in general, or subsist almost entirely on coffee and protein bars during the day. Your blood sugar should stay at a stasis point for the majority of the day, because if it soars and then crashes, you will feel it as a mood swing.

This blood sugar roller coaster makes PMS (and associated mood swings) worse, too. When your liver spends all its time and energy coping with crazy blood sugar shifts, its ability to detoxify your body and process and eliminate excess hormones can be impaired, which leads back to—you guessed it—more imbalanced hormones.

GUT HEALTH. A well-functioning, diverse microbiome—the millions of microbes that line your digestive system—is critical for stable mood. It's estimated that 90 percent of the serotonin in the body is made in the gut, and certain bacteria in the gut are crucial for making serotonin. And more serotonin equals a better mood.

MICRONUTRIENT DEFICIENCIES. If you have a history of overexercising, restricting calories, cutting out food groups, or drinking lots of caffeine and alcohol, or if you have taken synthetic birth control, your micronutrient tank may be depleted—leaving your body and brain missing key building blocks for stable moods.

Now, how can you use food to balance hormones and help support a stable mood? Be kind to your microbiome by avoiding the white stuff (sugar, flour, and dairy) and including small amounts of probiotic-rich foods like kimchi and sauerkraut in your diet. Taking a high-quality probiotic can also help—and bone broth is great, too, if you aren't vegetarian or vegan.

> YOUR BLOOD SUGAR
> SHOULD STAY AT A STASIS
> POINT FOR THE MAJORITY
> OF THE DAY, BECAUSE
> IF IT SOARS AND THEN
> CRASHES, YOU WILL FEEL
> IT AS A MOOD SWING.

To get your micronutrient levels back on track, seek out robust levels of vitamins B, D, and K, omega-3 fatty acids, and magnesium.

+ Grass-fed beef and salmon are good sources of vitamin B_6; vegetarians can get B_6 from spinach and chickpeas.

+ As for vitamin D and omega-3s, salmon and small oily fish like anchovies are good whole-food sources of both.

+ Get your vitamin K, or fat-soluble vitamins, from dark leafy greens and cruciferous veggies like broccoli, cauliflower, and Brussels sprouts.

+ And don't forget that dark chocolate is a good source of magnesium! So you can definitely keep that mood-booster on your list.

—ALISA VITTI,
HHC, AADP

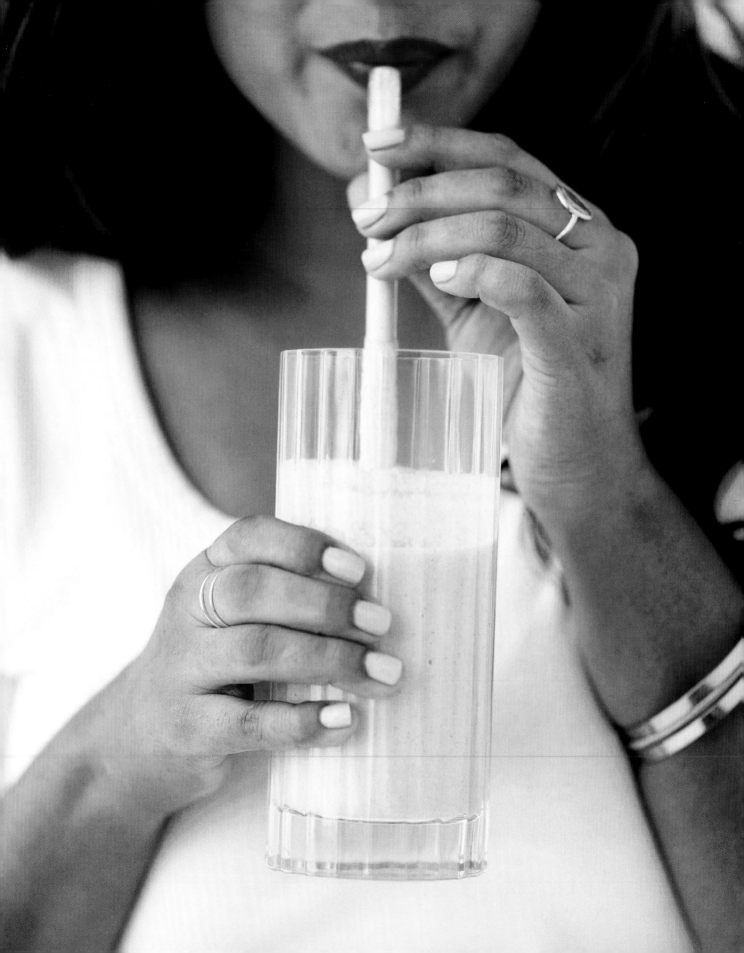

"The world of wellness can be daunting for people—so many superfoods, so little time," says Rachel Drori, CEO of subscription meal service Daily Harvest. "I believe that organic, plant-based food should be just as convenient as grabbing a protein bar." With this recipe, you mimic the aromatic spiciness of chai without having to buy a concentrate or brew tea ahead of time. How's that for convenience? Just another step toward an easier (and yummier) life.

CHAI + COCONUT SMOOTHIE

Serves 1

1 cup cauliflower florets

½ cup coconut meat

1 or 2 dates, such as Medjool or Deglet Noor

1 cup nondairy milk

¼ teaspoon grated fresh ginger, or ⅛ teaspoon ground ginger

¼ teaspoon ground cinnamon

¼ teaspoon ground cardamom

¼ teaspoon freshly ground black pepper

Pinch of pink Himalayan salt

1. In a high-speed blender, combine the cauliflower, coconut, date (use 2 dates if you prefer a sweeter smoothie), nondairy milk, ginger, cinnamon, cardamom, pepper, and salt. Blend until smooth.

2. Pour into a glass and enjoy.

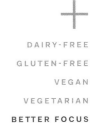

DAIRY-FREE

GLUTEN-FREE

VEGAN

VEGETARIAN

BETTER FOCUS

Basically, all you need to know is that Emmanuelle Sawko is a true Parisian and a real tastemaker (pun definitely intended) when it comes to food and aesthetics. This blue bowl (Emma's favorite color) reflects the free spirit you'll find inside her Wild & the Moon cafés (with locations in New York, Paris, and Dubai), which she describes as a lifestyle movement created by a tribe of food lovers, chefs, nutritionists, and naturopaths in France. "The philosophy at my café is based on the simple belief that food should be good for you, good for the planet, and delicious," says Emma. Peep the takeaway tip for puffing your quinoa—à la stovetop popcorn!

BLUE MAGIC SMOOTHIE BOWL

Serves 1

1½ cups sliced frozen banana
(about 2 medium)

1 cup frozen pineapple

1 cup coconut milk

½ teaspoon blue spirulina powder

TOPPINGS

1 tablespoon puffed quinoa,
store-bought or homemade
(recipe follows)

¼ cup fresh or frozen blueberries

1 small kiwi, peeled and sliced

1 teaspoon unsweetened
shredded coconut

+

DAIRY-FREE

GLUTEN-FREE

LOW-FODMAP

LOW-INFLAMMATION

VEGAN

VEGETARIAN

BETTER DIGESTION

BETTER SKIN

1. In a high-speed blender, combine the banana, pineapple, coconut milk, and spirulina. Blend until completely smooth.

2. Pour the smoothie mixture into a bowl and top with the puffed quinoa, blueberries, kiwi slices, and coconut. Serve cold.

PUFFED QUINOA

½ cup uncooked quinoa

1. Heat a small pot over high heat for 10 minutes. Add just enough quinoa to cover the bottom in a single layer (you may not need all the quinoa). Cover and shake vigorously until the quinoa starts popping rapidly, which will happen very quickly since the pot will be very hot. Remove the pot from the heat, continuing to shake. Crack the lid slightly, lifting it away from your face, to allow some steam to escape, then replace the lid fully and shake until the popping slows down to infrequent bursts.

2. Immediately pour the puffed quinoa onto a rimmed baking sheet and spread it into an even layer. Let cool completely before using. Store in an airtight container in the refrigerator for up to 1 week.

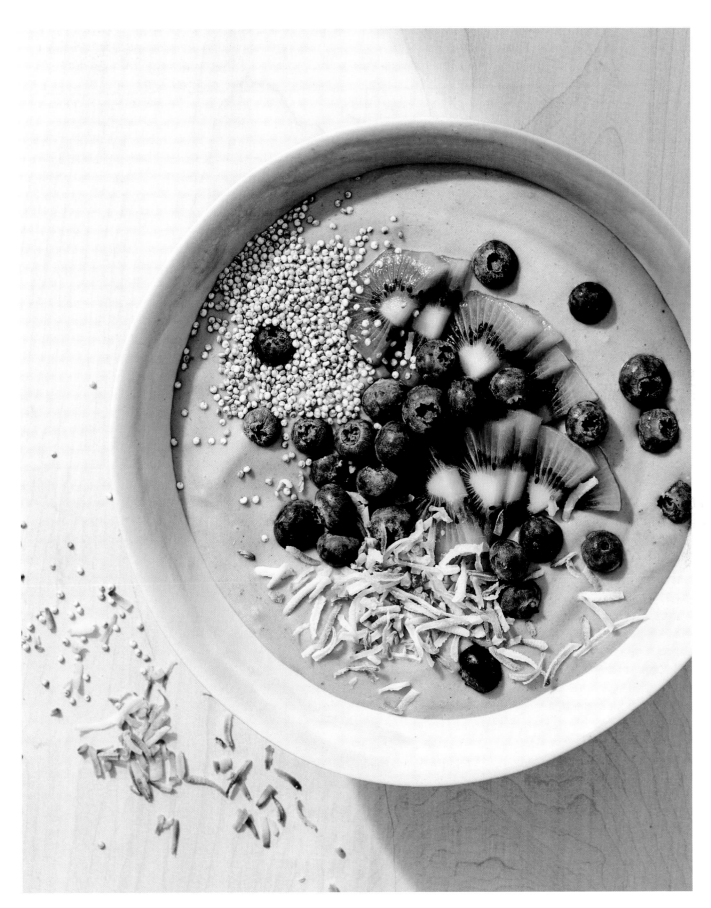

LIGHT
FARE

When she's not filming *Top Chef*, Padma Lakshmi tends to take a break from rich, decadent cuisine in favor of plant-based meals. "I use spices and fresh herbs in all my cooking, to add flavor and nuance without any added calories or fat," says the food expert, model, actress, and best-selling author. This dish is her attempt to re-create the flavors of Istanbul after encountering an eggplant dish in a trattoria on her way to see the Blue Mosque. It's an ideal mixture of sweet, salty, creamy, and spicy, and best served straight from the skin.

BAHARAT-SPICED EGGPLANT
WITH CHERRY TOMATOES + YOGURT

Serves 4

2 large eggplants

5 tablespoons extra-virgin olive oil

Kosher salt and freshly ground black pepper

2 medium yellow onions, diced

2 garlic cloves, minced

2 serrano peppers, minced

2 tablespoons baharat (see Tip)

½ teaspoon lime zest

2 to 3 tablespoons fresh lime juice (from about 1½ limes)

½ cup yogurt

1 cup cherry tomatoes, halved

4 tablespoons chopped fresh parsley

1. Preheat the oven to 425°F. Line a baking sheet with aluminum foil.

2. Halve each eggplant lengthwise. Score the insides of the eggplant flesh in a crosshatch pattern and place on the prepared baking sheet. Brush lightly with olive oil and season with salt and black pepper. Roast for about 45 minutes, or until fork-tender.

3. Meanwhile, heat 3 tablespoons of the oil in a large sauté pan over medium heat. When it shimmers, add the onions and cook, stirring occasionally, until golden brown, about 10 minutes. Taste and season with salt. Add the garlic, serranos, and baharat and cook for 2 minutes more, or until soft.

4. In a small bowl, stir together the lime zest and lime juice.

5. Transfer each roasted eggplant half to a plate. Divide the lime mixture over the tops. Add the onion mixture, dividing it evenly, and dress with the yogurt. Add ¼ cup of the cherry tomatoes and 1 tablespoon of the parsley to each. Serve.

GLUTEN-FREE

LOW-INFLAMMATION

PALEO

VEGETARIAN

BETTER MOOD

BETTER SLEEP

Tip: Baharat is a warm Middle Eastern spice blend that can be found in the spice aisle at grocery stores or online.

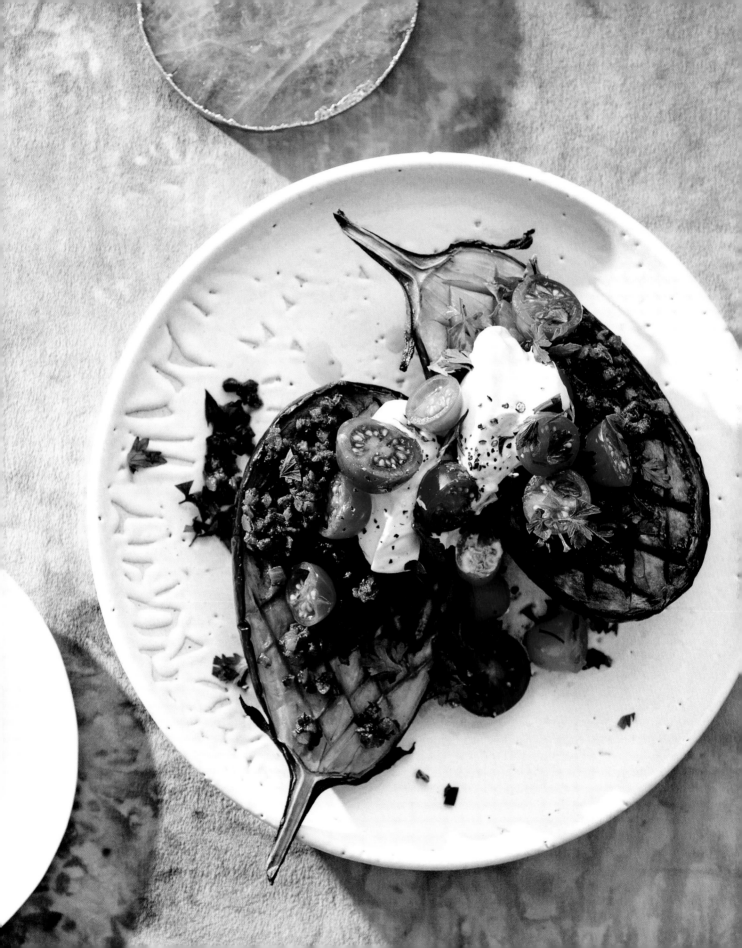

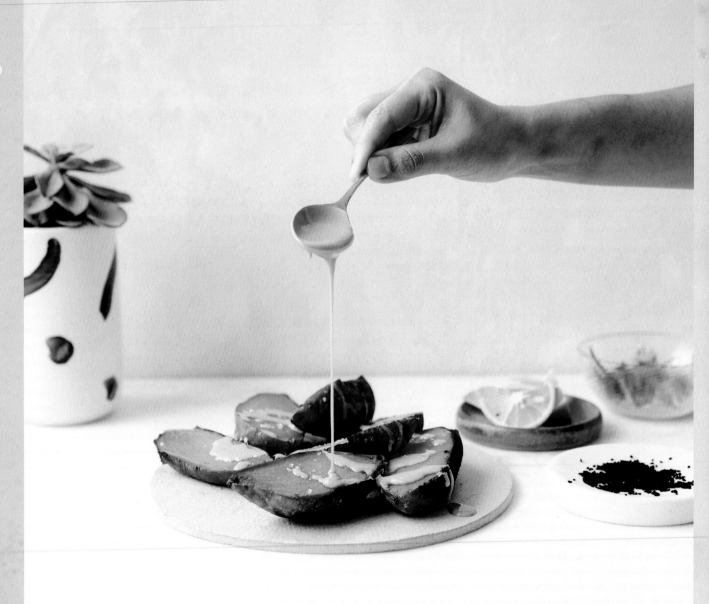

"I eat an obscene quantity of vegetables," says Julia Sherman, creator of Salad for President, an evolving publishing project that draws a meaningful connection between food, art, and everyday obsessions. (In other words, salad connoisseurs: Julia is making veggie love into an *art form*.) In this recipe, she keeps it simple—and delicious—with super-nutritious sweet potatoes and healthy fats in the form of tahini, for a dish that'll wow the crowd at your next BBQ. Don't have access to a gas flame or grill? Skip the first step and proceed without the char. "It's most important to remember not to take it all too seriously," Julia advises.

BARBECUED SWEET POTATO
WITH TAHINI DRIZZLE

Serves 4

4 small sweet potatoes, roasted or boiled

Sea salt

¼ cup tahini

4 teaspoons olive oil

¾ teaspoon nigella seeds (see Tip)

2 scallions, white and tender light-green parts only, sliced lengthwise as thinly as possible

Fresh lemon juice (optional)

1. Using metal tongs, and working with one at a time, hold the sweet potatoes over a low flame on your stovetop until the skin begins to char, rotating the potato to char it evenly all around. Transfer to a plate and repeat with the remaining potatoes.

2. Halve the charred potatoes lengthwise and season the inside of each with a generous pinch of salt. Arrange them on a serving dish and drizzle with the tahini. If the tahini is too thick to drizzle, thin it with water, 1 teaspoon at a time, stirring until desired consistency is reached. Drizzle the potatoes with the olive oil, then sprinkle the nigella seeds and scallions over the top. Finish with a squeeze of fresh lemon juice, if desired, and serve.

Tip: If you'd like, sub in cumin seeds—toast them in a small, dry skillet until fragrant, then transfer them to a small plate and let cool. Crush the seeds before adding them to the recipe in place of the nigella.

+

DAIRY-FREE

GLUTEN-FREE

LOW-INFLAMMATION

PALEO

VEGAN

VEGETARIAN

BETTER DIGESTION

BETTER ENERGY

BETTER MOOD

Guru Jagat—who has made the once underground practice of Kundalini yoga accessible to a young (celeb-heavy) audience—adapted this recipe based on her yogic research. With protein, bioavailable minerals and vitamins, and digestion-friendly spices, these pancakes have become a go-to meal. "Digestive metabolism is highly impactful on how you enjoy your body and experience your day," says the founder of RA MA Institute for Applied Yogic Science & Technology. The spiritual superstar stresses that for the pancakes to work their magic, you should stick to this alchemical low-heat timing of thirty minutes to preserve the nutrients.

JALAPEÑO PANCAKES

Makes 4 pancakes

½ cup bran

½ cup chickpea flour

1 (2-inch) piece fresh ginger, grated

3 tablespoons finely chopped cauliflower

2 small jalapeños, finely chopped

Oregano seeds

Crushed red pepper flakes

Coconut aminos

Kosher salt and freshly ground black pepper

Olive oil, for frying

Vegan sour cream, for serving (optional)

\+

DAIRY-FREE

GLUTEN-FREE

KETOGENIC

LOW-INFLAMMATION

PALEO

VEGAN

VEGETARIAN

BETTER DIGESTION

BETTER FOCUS

1. In a large bowl, stir together the bran, chickpea flour, ginger, cauliflower, and jalapeños and season with oregano seeds, red pepper flakes, coconut aminos, salt, and black pepper to taste. While stirring, add ¾ cup water and stir to create a thick batter (it should be thick enough to give some resistance as you stir, but still easy enough to move your spoon through without a lot of effort).

2. Heat ¼ inch of olive oil in a large skillet over low heat. When it shimmers, working in batches, use a ¼-cup measure to scoop the mixture into the pan and form 4 pancakes. Cook for 15 minutes on each side, until golden and cooked through.

3. Serve warm, with a dollop of vegan sour cream on top, if desired.

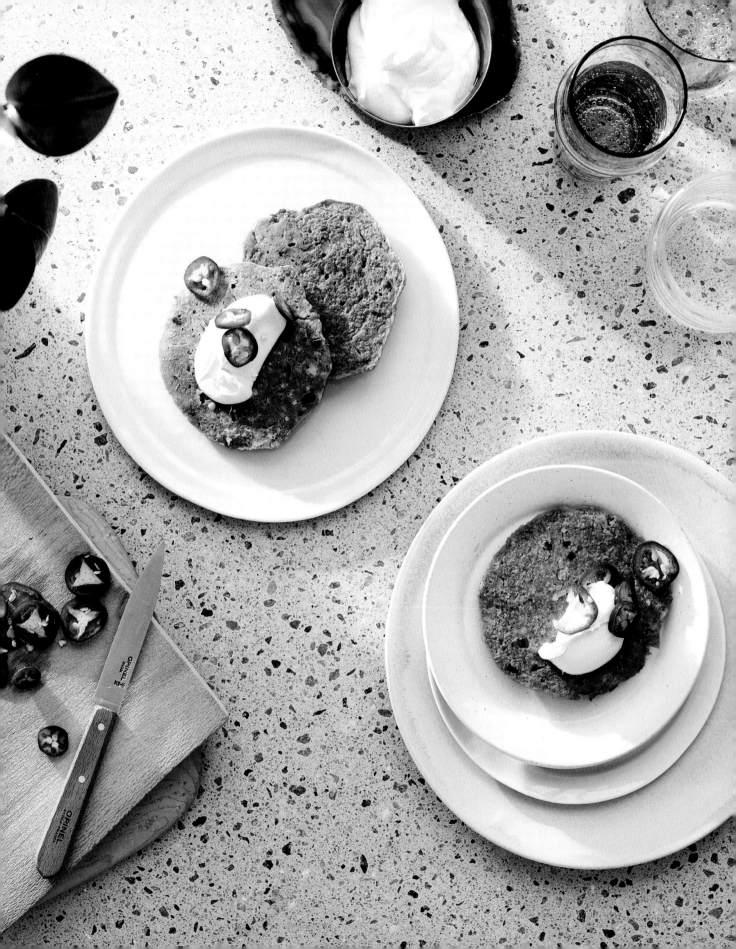

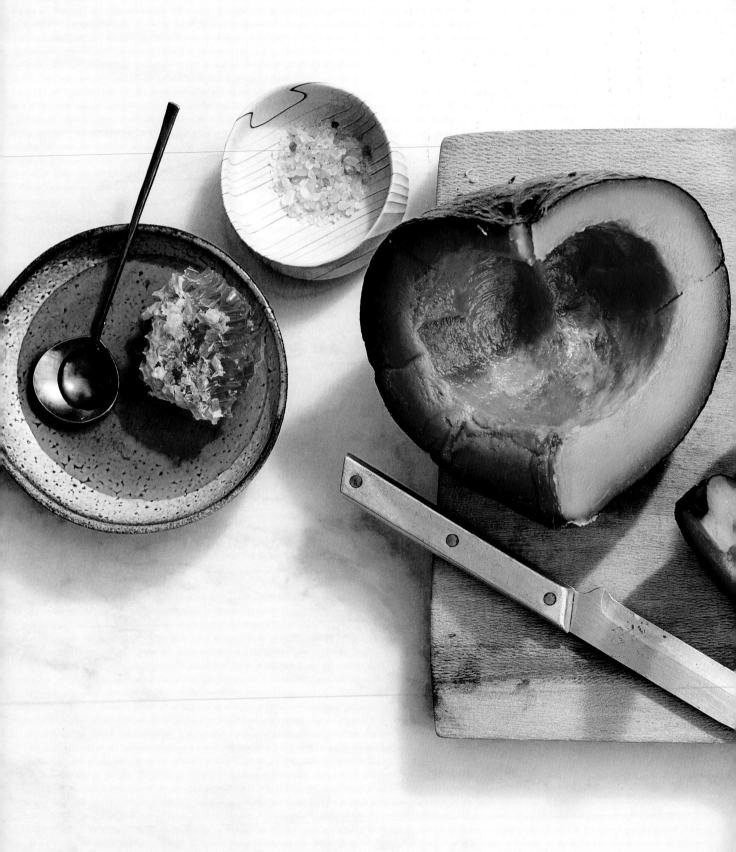

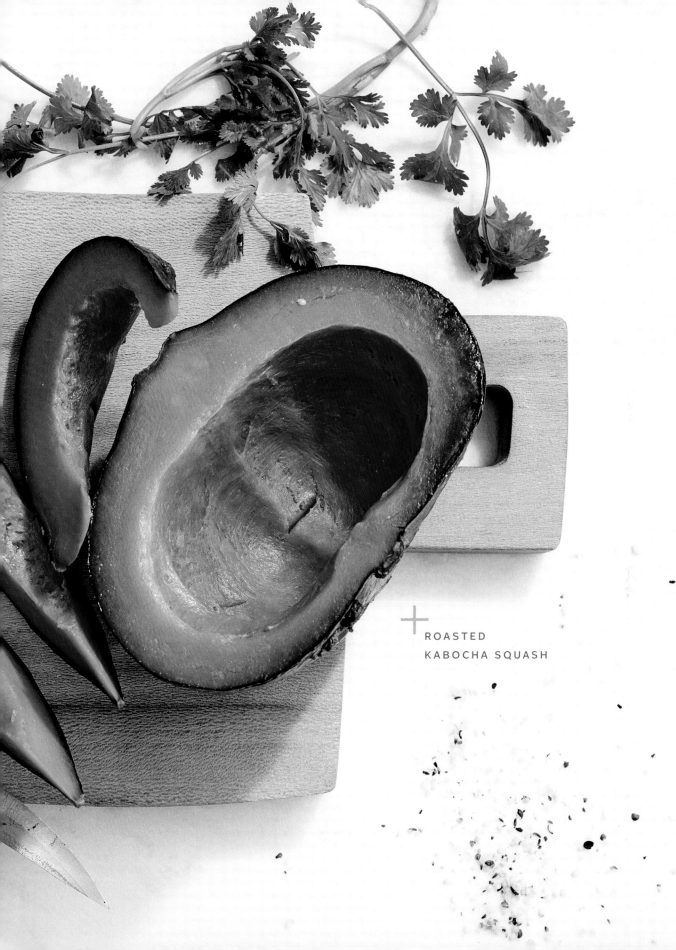

+ ROASTED
KABOCHA SQUASH

Fitness phenomenon Taryn Toomey is renowned for the (sweaty) soul journey she takes her students on in The Class, a cathartic mind-body fitness experience that definitely nudges you out of your personal comfort zone. It's a deeply intuitive process, and when Taryn's fueling up outside the studio, she stays tuned to what her body needs and feeds it accordingly. "I am a fan of eating real, whole foods that are grown from the earth or found in the sea," she says. "If I need grounding, I'll eat dense foods, like kabocha squash or root vegetables." This recipe is nutrient-dense, filling, and, best of all, easy to whip up, no matter how tired you are post–sweat session.

ROASTED KABOCHA SQUASH

Serves 2

1 small kabocha squash

1 tablespoon coconut oil

Pink Himalayan salt

1 tablespoon raw honey

1 tablespoon hemp seeds

½ teaspoon ground cinnamon

Handful of fresh cilantro leaves (optional)

1. Preheat the oven to 425°F. Line a baking sheet with aluminum foil.

2. Scrub the squash and dry it completely. Halve it lengthwise and scrape out the seeds. Smear the coconut oil all over the skin of the squash and season with salt.

3. Arrange the squash cut-side down on the prepared baking sheet. Roast for 30 minutes, or until softened. Remove from the oven and let the squash cool slightly, then cut it into 2-inch pieces.

4. Drizzle the honey over the top and sprinkle with the hemp seeds and cinnamon. Garnish with the cilantro leaves, if desired, and serve.

DAIRY-FREE

GLUTEN-FREE

LOW-INFLAMMATION

PALEO

VEGETARIAN

BETTER SEX

BETTER SKIN

KERRILYNN
PAMER

+

CINDY
DIPRIMA
MORISSE

"We live by the motto that beauty is wellness—and wellness is beauty," say Kerrilynn Pamer and Cindy DiPrima Morisse, founders of CAP Beauty, the high-vibrational boutique that those in the know are obsessed with. The duo applies this philosophy to all aspects of their lives, including food: "Our take on gazpacho is a—not surprisingly—up-leveled, hippie-inspired affair." Taking a cue from Gingersnap's Organic—the plant-based New York restaurant that inspired a cult following before shutting its doors in 2017—they add chipotle chile and nutritional yeast to turn traditional gazpacho into a smoky-tasting delicious soup.

GAZPACHO SUPERIOR

Serves 4

5 tomatoes, coarsely chopped (4 to 5 cups)

1 large cucumber, peeled and coarsely chopped

1 shallot

1 sun-dried tomato, or to taste

Pink Himalayan salt and freshly ground black pepper

1 tablespoon nutritional yeast

½ teaspoon chile de árbol

½ teaspoon smoky chile flakes (chipotle works well)

1 teaspoon pimentón flakes or smoked paprika

1 teaspoon apple cider vinegar

1 tablespoon olive oil

1. In a high-speed blender, combine the chopped tomatoes, cucumber, shallot, and sun-dried tomato. Season generously with salt and pepper, then blend until smooth enough to stir with a spoon and thoroughly combined. Add the nutritional yeast, chile de árbol, chile flakes, pimentón flakes, and vinegar and blend for 1 minute more, or until creamy (or until the desired consistency is reached).

2. Divide the gazpacho among four bowls, drizzle with the olive oil, and finish with salt. Serve.

Tip: Add an ice cube for a refreshing, extra-chilled summertime soup.

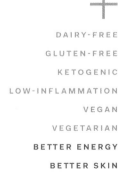

DAIRY-FREE

GLUTEN-FREE

KETOGENIC

LOW-INFLAMMATION

VEGAN

VEGETARIAN

BETTER ENERGY

BETTER SKIN

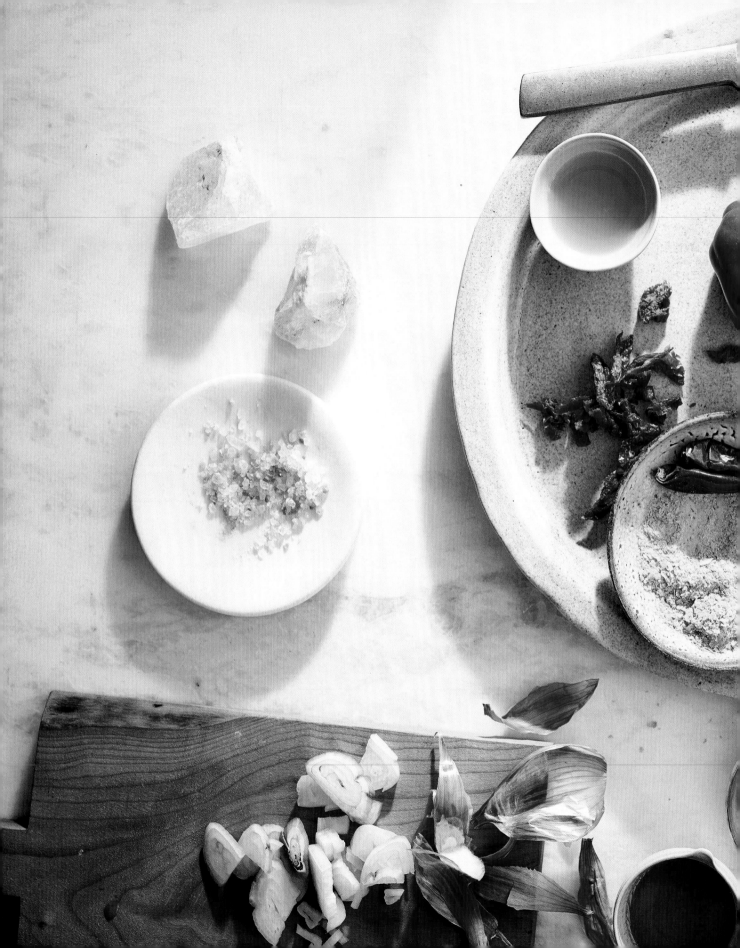

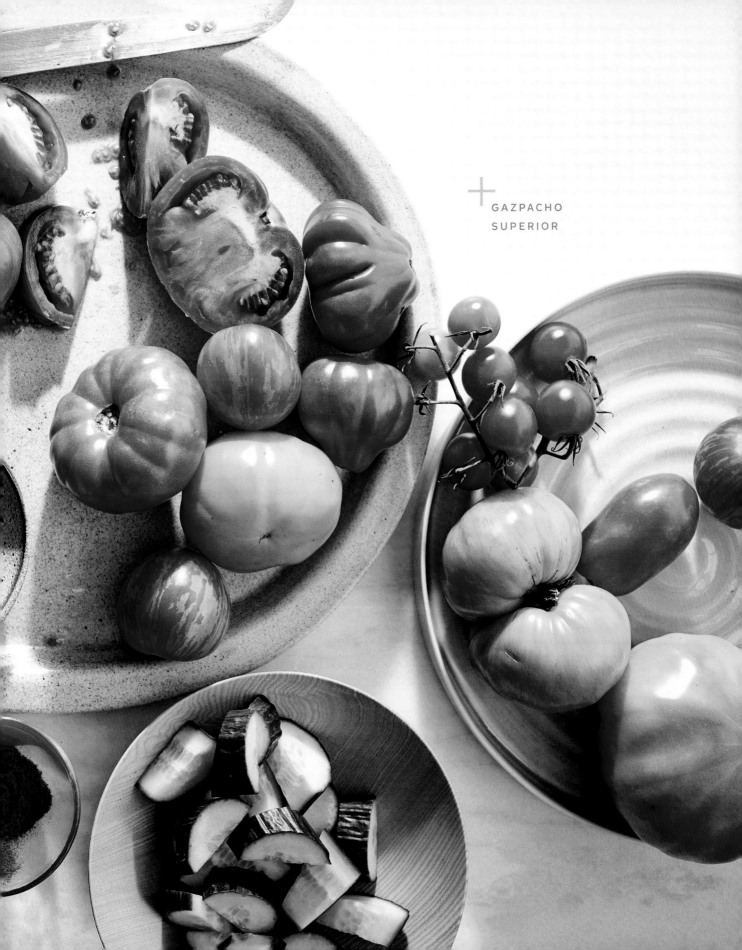

GAZPACHO
SUPERIOR

You probably know Ali Maffucci best for her culinary brand, Inspiralized (and the spiralized veggie craze she helped kick off), and the blogger and three-time cookbook author continues to be on the lookout for innovative ways to make over mealtime. "By using real, whole foods creatively, we hit the trifecta: Food is fun, delicious, and healthy," she says. This recipe is a better-for-you take on Italian American "parmigiana" dishes (breaded meat or vegetables topped with marinara sauce, Parmesan, and mozzarella), which Ali promises never disappoints. "You get the same flavors of those dishes, but the veggie version is better nutritionally and lower in cholesterol."

CAULIFLOWER-PARMESAN BITES

Serves 6

Coconut oil spray

½ cup unsweetened almond milk

¼ cup grated Parmesan cheese, plus more for garnish

½ cup almond flour

2 teaspoons garlic powder

2 teaspoons onion powder

1 teaspoon dried oregano

¼ teaspoon crushed red pepper flakes, plus more for garnish

Kosher salt and freshly ground black pepper

1 large head cauliflower, broken into florets

½ cup prepared marinara sauce

1 cup shredded mozzarella cheese

2 fresh basil leaves, very thinly sliced

1. Preheat the oven to 450°F. Line a baking sheet with parchment paper and coat the parchment with coconut oil spray.

2. In a large bowl, whisk together the almond milk, Parmesan, almond flour, garlic powder, onion powder, oregano, red pepper flakes, and ½ cup water. Season with salt and black pepper. Dredge the cauliflower florets through the mixture, coating them well and patting the mixture into the crevices of the cauliflower. Place the coated florets on the prepared baking sheet and bake for 20 minutes. Flip and bake for 20 minutes more, or until the cauliflower is fork-tender and golden brown on the outside.

3. Remove the cauliflower from the oven and turn the broiler to high. Top each cauliflower piece with a dollop of marinara sauce and some mozzarella. Return the pan to the oven and broil for 2 to 3 minutes, until the mozzarella begins bubbling.

4. Remove and immediately garnish with more Parmesan, the basil, and red pepper flakes. Transfer the cauliflower to a serving platter and spear each floret with a toothpick. Serve immediately.

GLUTEN-FREE

VEGETARIAN

BETTER FOCUS

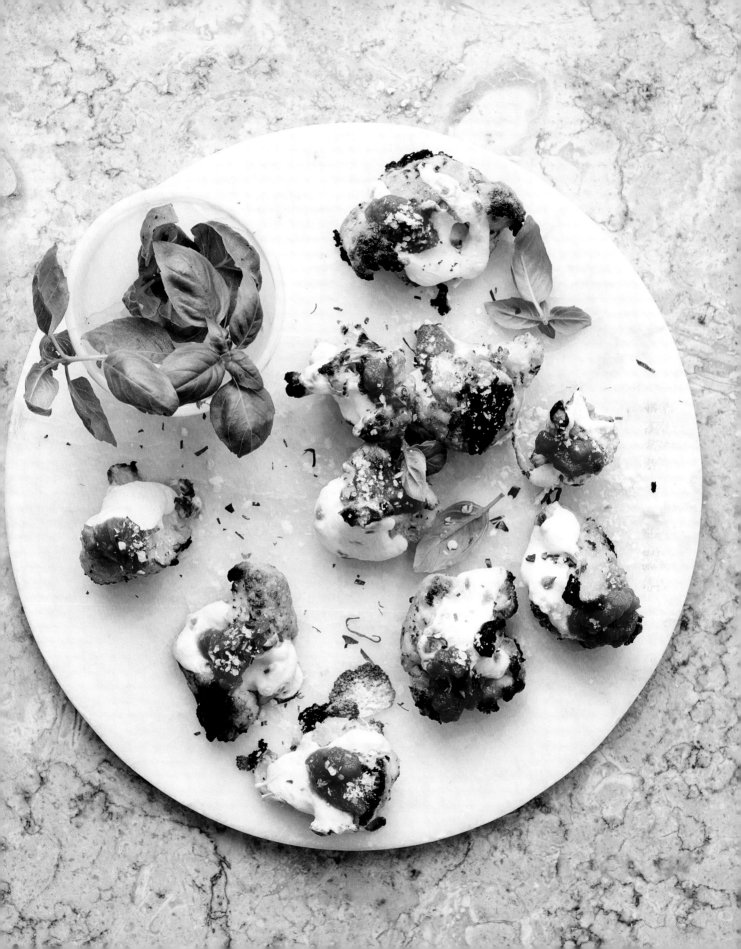

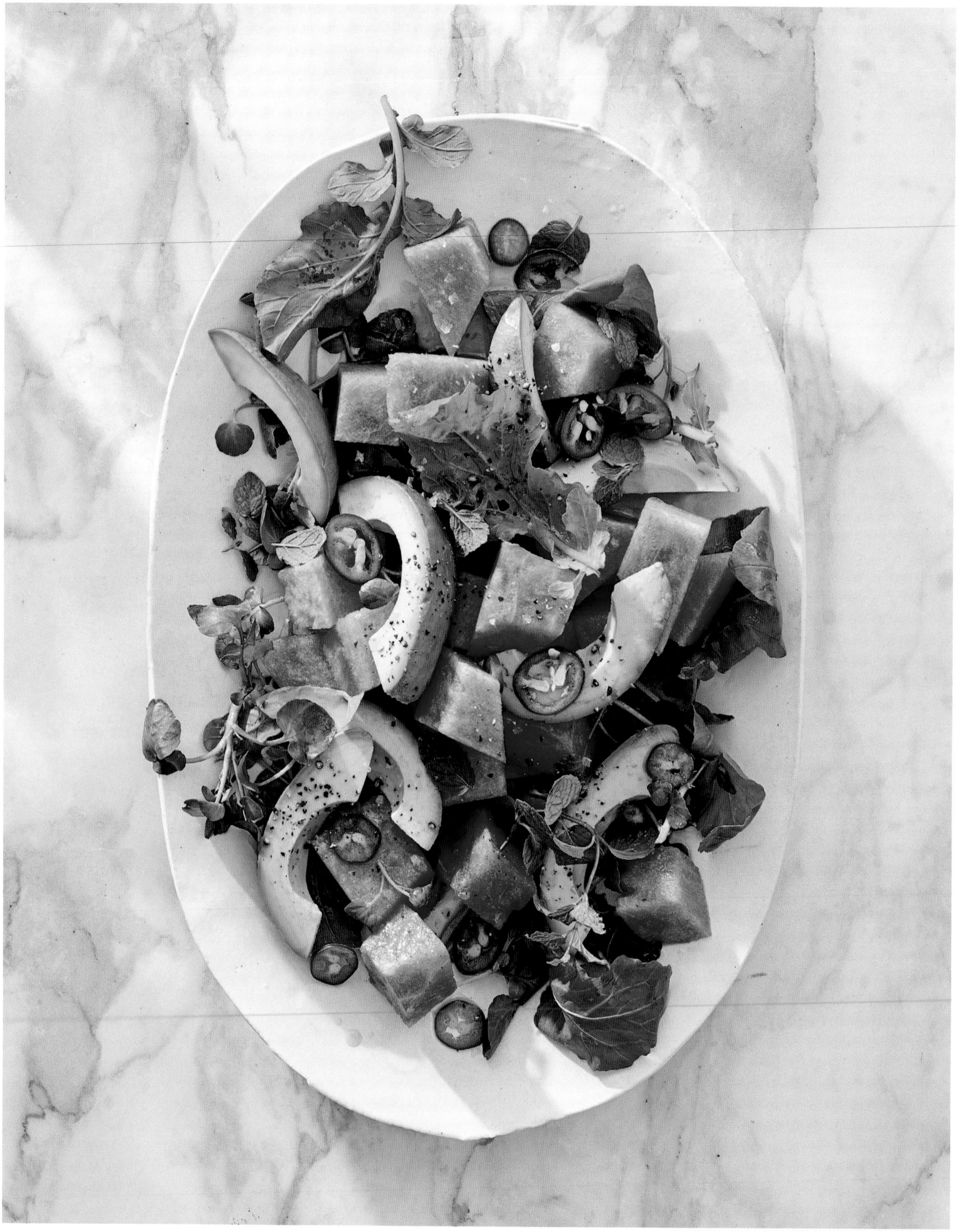

This fruit-forward dish came to Well+Good cofounder Melisse Gelula on a hot day, inspired by the simple salads she has eaten abroad. "In Australia, sweet and spicy flavors more typically accentuate produce, rather than cloying American salad dressing," she says. Melisse makes this light fare for friends often, using grapefruit juice as a dressing free of needless added sugar. "Every time, they act like they've never had watermelon and avocado before," she says. "Super simple can totally get rave reviews."

SPICY WATERMELON SALAD

Serves 2

FOR THE DRESSING

1 small grapefruit (preferably red)

1 small jalapeño, seeded and thinly sliced

Pinch of sea salt

FOR THE SALAD

1 small bunch watercress

1 small bunch arugula

2 cups coarsely cubed watermelon

1 medium avocado, pitted, peeled, and sliced

4 mint sprigs, coarsely chopped

1 tablespoon olive oil

Fresh lime juice

Slivered almonds (optional)

Pink Himalayan salt

1. Make the dressing. Roll the grapefruit back and forth on a cutting board, then cut it into quarters. Use your hands to squeeze the juice of the grapefruit into a small bowl. Add the jalapeño and sea salt. Set aside for at least 20 minutes to allow the heat of the pepper to infuse the grapefruit.

2. Meanwhile, make the salad. On a large serving platter, arrange the watercress and arugula so they cover most of the platter. Add the watermelon and layer the avocado slices on top.

3. Gently strain the grapefruit dressing over the salad, reserving the jalapeños, being sure to cover the watermelon and avocado but not to drown the watercress. Place the jalapeños around the edges of the platter.

4. Sprinkle the mint over the top and finish with a drizzle of olive oil, a squeeze of lime juice, the almonds (if using), and a pinch or two of pink Himalayan salt. Serve immediately.

Tip: Arranging the jalapeños around the edges of the platter allows eaters who can't take the heat to enjoy the whole dish.

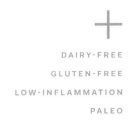

DAIRY-FREE

GLUTEN-FREE

LOW-INFLAMMATION

PALEO

VEGAN

VEGETARIAN

BETTER SKIN

"This salad is one of my faves to whip up in the summer," says Eden Grinshpan, the Canadian Israeli chef of DEZ in New York City's Nolita. Traditionally panzanella is made by taking stale bread, drenching it in vinaigrette, and tossing it with onions and tomatoes, but Eden gives it a Middle Eastern twist, adding sumac, a spice with lots of zing and lemony flavor. "A rule to follow is, 'What grows together, goes together,'" says the food television personality. Her words couldn't be more true—as you'll see, the tanginess of the tomatoes and the sweet peaches are a dreamy, delicious partnership indeed.

SUMAC PITA, TOMATO + PEACH PANZANELLA

Serves 4

FOR THE TOASTED SUMAC PITA

3 tablespoons extra-virgin olive oil

1 to 2 pitas, torn into bite-size pieces

1 tablespoon ground sumac

Pinch of sea salt

FOR THE VINAIGRETTE

Juice of ½ lemon (about 1 tablespoon)

1 teaspoon honey

1 teaspoon red wine vinegar

6 tablepsoons olive oil

Kosher salt and freshly ground black pepper

DAIRY-FREE

LOW-INFLAMMATION

PALEO

VEGETARIAN

BETTER FOCUS

FOR THE SALAD

2 cups coarsely chopped heirloom tomatoes (different sizes and colors encouraged)

½ cup roughly torn fresh flat-leaf parsley, plus a handful of parsley leaves for garnish

½ cup roughly torn fresh mint, plus several whole mint leaves for garnish

1 peach, pitted and thinly sliced

½ red onion, thinly sliced

1 teaspoon ground sumac (optional)

1. Make the pita. Heat the oil in a medium skillet over high heat. When it shimmers, add the pitas and reduce the heat to medium-low. Season with the sumac and salt, then cook, stirring occasionally and flipping to cook both sides, for 10 to 15 minutes, until golden and crisp all over. Transfer the pitas to a paper towel–lined plate to drain.

2. Make the vinaigrette. In a medium bowl, whisk together the lemon juice, honey, and vinegar. While whisking, slowly drizzle in the olive oil and whisk until emulsified. Season with salt and pepper.

3. Assemble the salad. In a large bowl, combine the tomatoes, parsley, mint, peach, red onion, and toasted pita. Pour over the vinaigrette and sprinkle with the sumac, if desired. Toss to coat thoroughly. Garnish with parsley and mint leaves and serve.

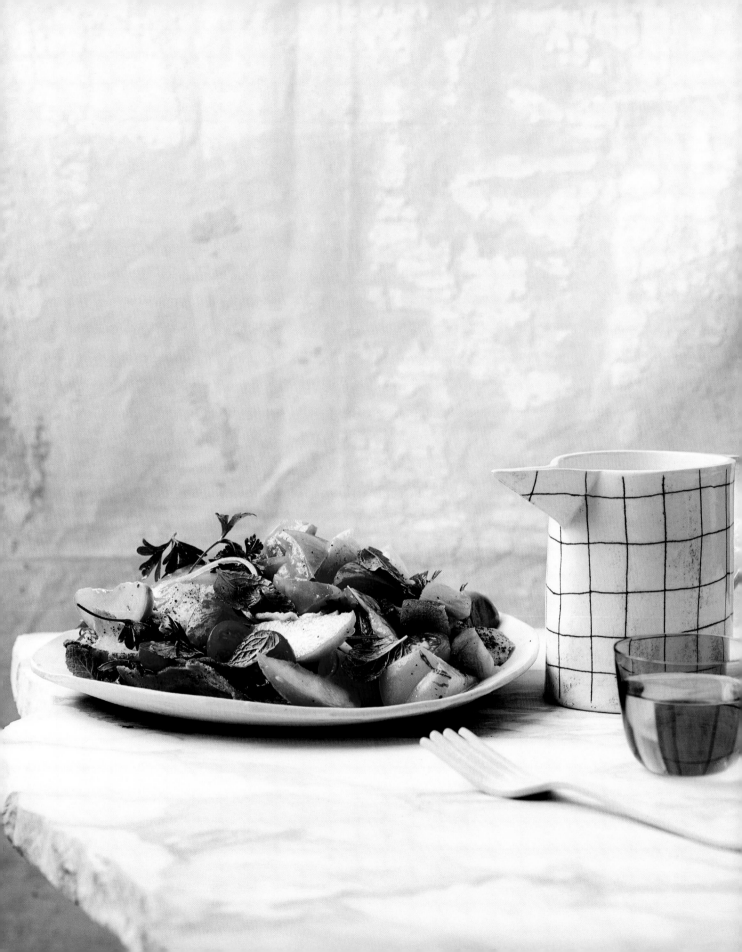

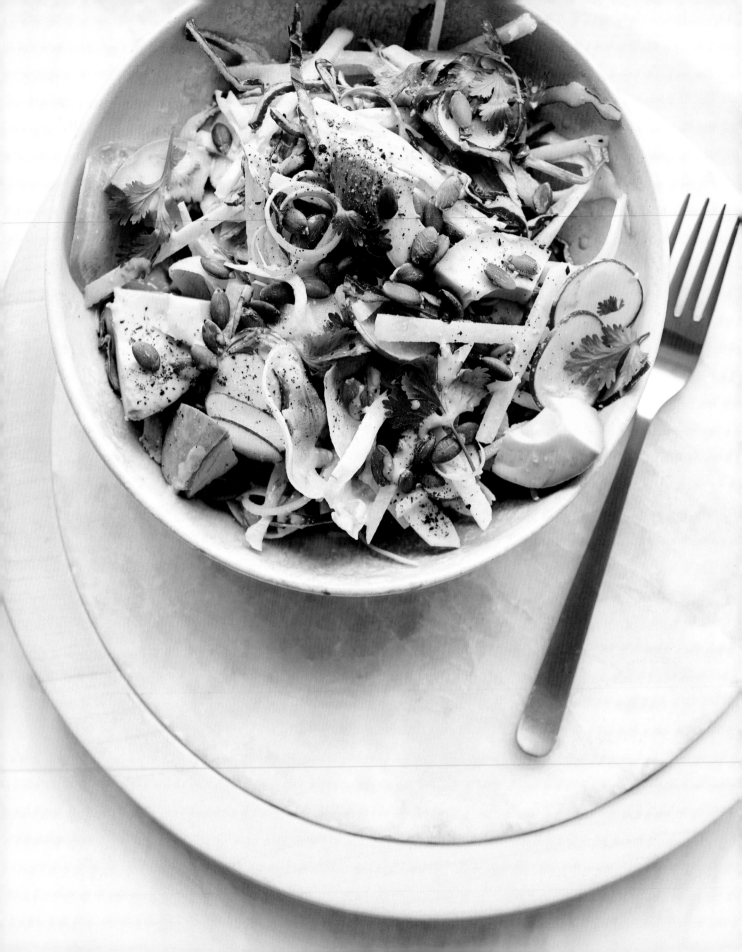

Amy Chaplin, the former executive chef at the renowned (though now sadly closed) vegan hot spot Angelica Kitchen in New York, is a James Beard Award–winning cookbook author, chef, teacher, and consultant. But mostly, she's a magician with veggies (just ask her famous clients like Natalie Portman and Liv Tyler). "My approach to food is inspired by nature and the healing benefits of whole food ingredients," she says. Jicama, the root vegetable star of this slaw, ups your fiber intake and adds some serious crunch. If you aren't in the mood for a creamy dressing, you can simply toss this slaw with fresh lime and orange (or tangerine!) juice and season to taste.

JICAMA SLAW

Serves 6

FOR THE DRESSING

Zest of 1 lime

3 tablespoons raw cashew butter

6 tablespoons fresh lime juice

1 tablespoon apple cider vinegar

1 small garlic clove, crushed

3 tablespoons extra-virgin olive oil or cold-pressed flaxseed oil

Sea salt

FOR THE SLAW

1 large jicama, peeled and cut into matchsticks (3 to 5 cups)

¼ medium red cabbage, thinly sliced (about 2 cups)

1 medium fennel bulb, cored and thinly sliced

2 watermelon radishes, shaved

3 red radishes, shaved

2 scallions, thinly sliced

Kosher salt

1 large avocado, pitted, peeled, and sliced

3 tablespoons pumpkin seeds, toasted

2 cups fresh cilantro leaves

1. Make the dressing. In a small bowl, stir together the lime zest, cashew butter, and 3 tablespoons of the lime juice until smooth. Stir in the remaining 3 tablespoons lime juice, the vinegar, and the garlic, then stir in the olive oil and season with sea salt. If the mixture is too thick, stir in water, a little at a time, until the desired consistency is reached.

2. Make the slaw. In a large bowl, toss the jicama, cabbage, fennel, both radishes, and scallions to combine.

3. Drizzle the dressing over the salad and toss again. Taste and season with kosher salt as needed. Arrange the avocado on top, sprinkle with the pumpkin seeds and cilantro, and serve.

+

DAIRY-FREE

GLUTEN-FREE

PALEO

VEGAN

VEGETARIAN

BETTER ENERGY

BETTER SKIN

"Some days you work out and eat your greens—other days are enjoyed in bed with pajamas and chocolate chip cookies," says Elisa Marshall. In other words, there are many ways to "veg out"—and when she's in the mood to do it with vitamins (as opposed to a fluffy duvet), Elisa, owner of Maman, a beautiful café, bakery, restaurant, and event space with locations in New York and Toronto, turns to this soup. Full of fragrant herbs and nutrient-dense mixed greens, "It feels like comfort in a bowl," she says.

GREEN HERB VELOUTÉ

Serves 2

1 tablespoon olive oil, plus more for drizzling

1 bunch scallions, thinly sliced

Sea salt

4 cups mixed greens, such as spinach, arugula, dandelion, and watercress, stemmed

Freshly ground black pepper

4 cups vegetable broth

¼ cup finely chopped fresh chives, plus more for garnish

1 tablespoon fresh mint leaves

¼ cup fresh flat-leaf parsley leaves

2 tablespoons fresh chervil or tarragon leaves

3 ounces brousse or other soft cheese, for garnish (optional)

1. Heat the olive oil in a large saucepan over medium heat. When it shimmers, add the scallions, season with salt, and cook until softened, 1 to 2 minutes. Add the mixed greens and season with salt and pepper. Pour in the broth, increase the heat to medium-high, and bring to a boil. Cook for 3 minutes, then add the chives, mint, parsley, and chervil and cook for about 1 minute, or until wilted.

2. Fill a large bowl with ice and set it nearby. Transfer the contents of the pot to a blender and blend until very smooth (or use an immersion blender to blend the mixture directly in the pot). Transfer the blended velouté to a medium metal bowl and set it over the bowl of ice to allow the chlorophyll to set, preserving the bright green color.

3. To serve, divide the velouté between two bowls, top with the cheese, if desired, and garnish with chives. Finish with a drizzle of olive oil.

GLUTEN-FREE

LOW-INFLAMMATION

VEGAN

VEGETARIAN

BETTER MOOD

BETTER SKIN

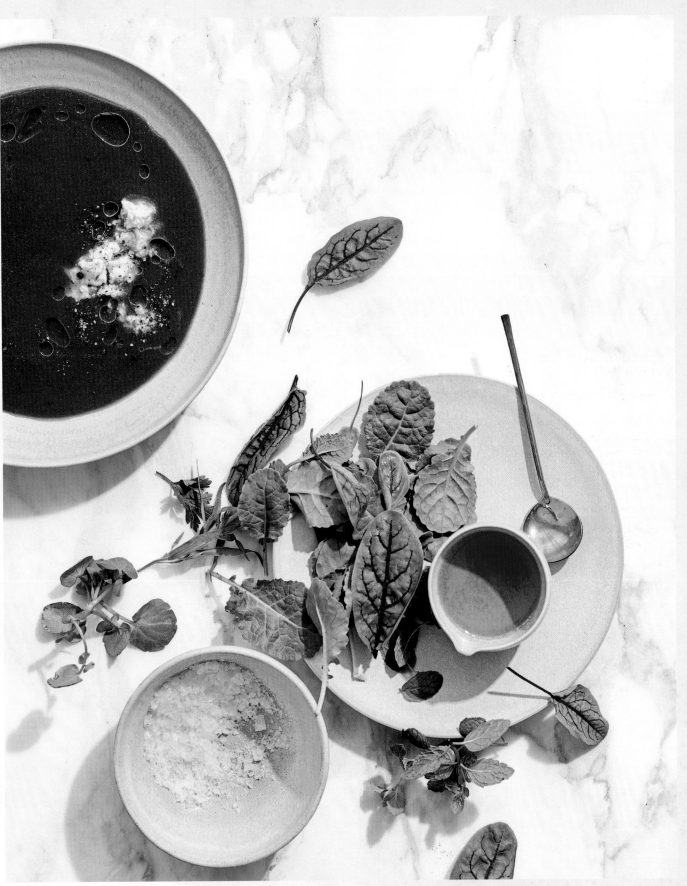

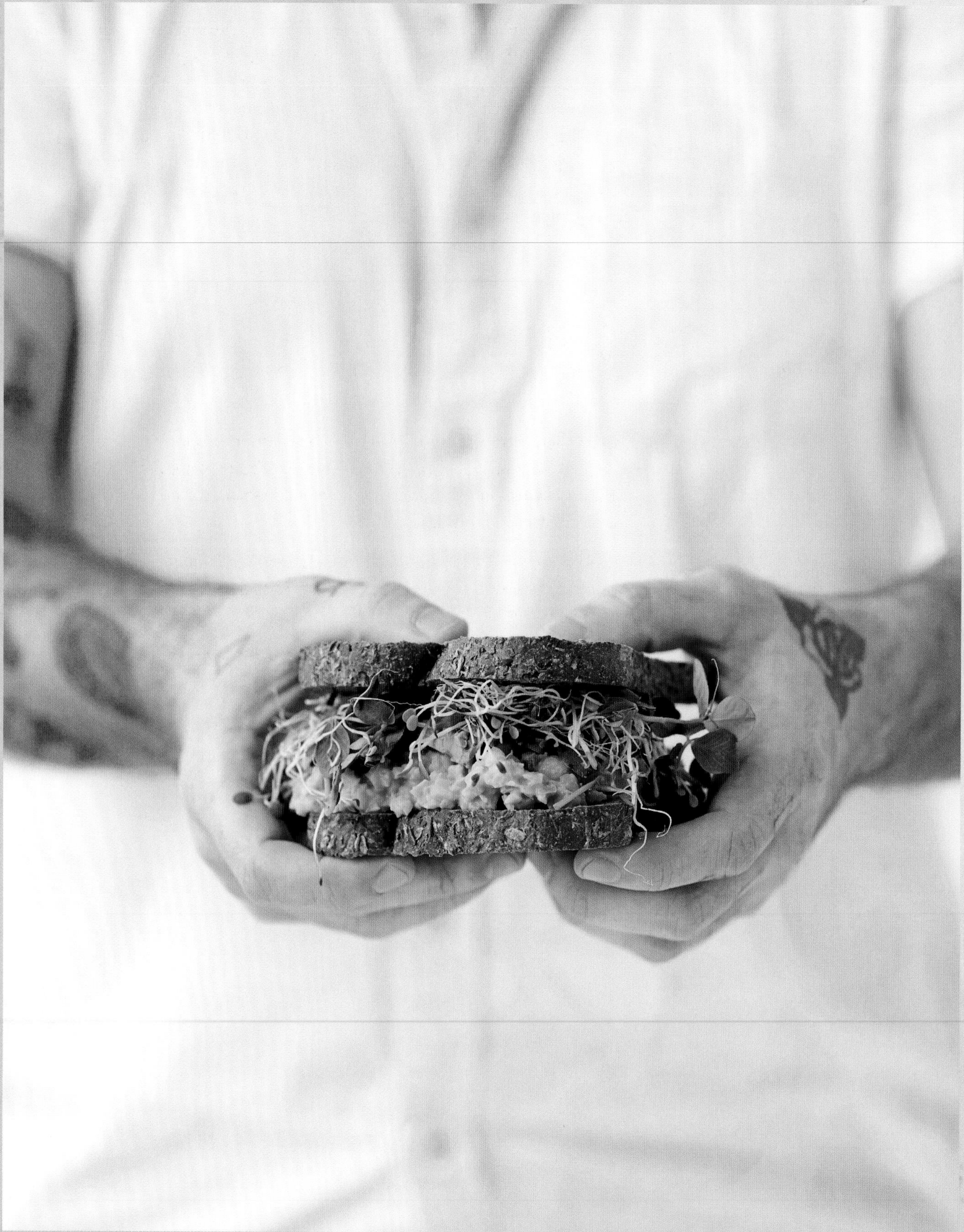

Beauty-ingredient activist (and literal rock star) Alexis Krauss has been a vegetarian for years, but she swears that giving up dairy was hands-down the absolute best thing she did for herself. "It took a lot of discipline and self-control at first, but now it feels so natural," says the cofounder of the ethical advocacy site Beauty Lies Truth and frontwoman of the pop duo Sleigh Bells. She found a yummy creaminess with this dish. Say good-bye to a sad desk lunch—this time-savvy recipe is even an option for morning meal-prepping.

CHICKPEA SALAD SANDWICH

Makes enough for 2 sandwiches

1 (15-ounce) can chickpeas, drained and rinsed

¼ cup vegan mayonnaise

1 tablespoon extra-virgin olive oil

Juice of 1 lemon (optional)

½ cup chopped celery

½ cup diced carrots

Dash of garlic powder

1 tablespoon nutritional yeast

1 teaspoon ground turmeric

Toasted sprouted bread

½ medium avocado, pitted, peeled, and sliced, for serving

Handful of alfalfa sprouts, for garnish

Pink Himalayan salt and freshly ground black pepper

1. In a food processor, combine the chickpeas, mayonnaise, olive oil, and lemon juice (if using). Pulse until the ingredients are broken down to a coarse texture and combined. The chickpeas should be lightly mashed, but still retain some shape.

2. Spoon the mixture into a medium bowl and add the celery, carrots, garlic powder, nutritional yeast, and turmeric. Stir with a wooden spoon until evenly mixed.

3. Spread the chickpea salad onto freshly toasted bread and layer on the avocado and some sprouts. Season with salt and pepper and enjoy.

4. Store any leftover chickpea salad in an airtight container in the refrigerator for up to 1 week.

+

DAIRY-FREE

LOW-INFLAMMATION

VEGAN

VEGETARIAN

BETTER MOOD

BETTER SLEEP

EAT FOR BETTER DIGESTION

When your digestion feels off, it can affect everything from your mood to your skin—not to mention causing symptoms like bloating, gas, heartburn, abdominal pain, constipation, and diarrhea. So how do you get a happy belly? With my patients, I've found that making these four diet and lifestyle changes is the best way to improve digestion and overall health.

NURTURE YOUR MICROBIOME. Consuming small amounts of fermented foods in your diet, like sauerkraut, kimchi, and kombucha, can promote high levels of healthy bacteria in your gut. These bacteria are important because they're involved in everything from helping to regulate your immune system, weight, and blood sugar to soothing irritable bowel syndrome. Prebiotic foods—those that feed your microbes—like artichokes, asparagus, garlic, onion, and oats are also essential. If you have specific digestive issues, you may also want to work with your doctor to find a high-quality medical-grade probiotic supplement that works for you. Gut health is *not* just a trend. New science on the gut microbiome is emerging every day.

CUT OUT SUGAR AND PROCESSED FOODS. Eating too much sugar in the form of processed foods can lead to an overgrowth of bad bacteria in the gut, which can crowd out the good bacteria and increase inflammation. Your body actually craves sugar more when your gut microbiome is unbalanced, so getting your gut health in check should help.

GUT HEALTH IS *NOT* JUST A TREND. NEW SCIENCE ON THE GUT MICROBIOME IS EMERGING EVERY DAY.

Eating protein and healthy fats at each meal will also help cut down on sugar cravings. And if you're going to eat carbohydrates, they should be in the form of whole foods like oats, quinoa, and sweet potatoes—not highly processed carbs like pasta and bread.

And to *really* root out the sweet stuff, beware of sneaky sources of added sugar, which you'll find listed on ingredient labels under names like "evaporated cane juice," "corn syrup," "glucose," "sucrose," "honey," "molasses," and "agave," among many others.

EAT MORE MINDFULLY. Raise your hand if you've ever eaten a salad at your desk, scarfed down oatmeal in the carpool line, or sat down for dinner in front of the TV. We all have. And chances are, you might not have felt so great afterward. That's because when you're not eating slowly and mindfully, you're probably not chewing properly. As you chew, saliva softens the food, making it easier to digest—if you swallow before the food is basically liquefied, the rest of your digestive system has to work harder to digest it, resulting in stomach discomfort.

EXPERIMENT WITH ELIMINATING CERTAIN FOODS. If you're eating all the right foods and still have GI issues, you might have a food sensitivity. Eliminating some foods from your diet and then reintroducing them one by one can help you uncover what's bothering you.

An elimination diet typically involves removing things like gluten, dairy, eggs, soy, corn, peanuts, and sugar or artificial sweeteners for at least thirty days—then slowly adding them back in and taking note of any symptoms that arise after each reintroduction. A doctor, health coach, or nutritionist can guide you through the process.

—ROBIN BERZIN, MD

Yoga It-girls Krissy Jones and Chloe Kernaghan came on the New York City scene back in 2015 with Sky Ting, their lofty oasis in Chinatown, and haven't stopped flexing since. The two have since expanded their animal-themed studio (think: giant giraffes and flamingo fun décor) to include multiple locations, a 200-hour teacher-training program, global retreats, and a new video platform, which made us wonder, *When do these bustling wellness entrepreneurs have time to eat at home?* "Easy assembly and a mix of raw foods, veggies, and grains is key," says Chloe. This bowl is a fusion of Chloe's lunch routine topped with a dressing that Krissy puts on (almost) everything.

QUINOA VEGGIE BOWL

Serves 1

1 large egg

1 teaspoon coconut oil

½ garlic clove, minced

1 cup chopped kale, Swiss chard, or spinach

Coarse sea salt

½ cup cooked sprouted quinoa

½ avocado, pitted and peeled

⅓ cup kimchi (cabbage, cucumber, or radish)

½ cup roasted mixed vegetables, such as sweet potato, Brussels sprouts, broccoli, and carrots (optional)

2 tablespoons Lemon Vinaigrette (recipe follows)

1 tablespoon toasted sesame seeds

Freshly ground black pepper

DAIRY-FREE

LOW-INFLAMMATION

VEGETARIAN

BETTER DIGESTION

BETTER ENERGY

BETTER SKIN

1. Bring a small pot of water to a boil over high heat. Fill a small bowl with ice and water and set it nearby. Gently lower the egg into the water and cook for exactly 6 minutes for a perfectly runny yolk (or cook longer, according to your preference). Drain the egg and plunge it into the ice water to stop the cooking. When cool enough to handle, peel the egg.

2. Melt the coconut oil in a small skillet over medium heat. When it shimmers, add the garlic and cook, stirring, until fragrant, about 1 minute. Add the kale and cook until wilted, about 2 minutes. Season with salt.

3. Place the quinoa in a shallow bowl. Top with the avocado, kimchi, cooked kale, and roasted vegetables (if using). Carefully slice the egg in half and arrange it on top. Drizzle with the vinaigrette and scatter the sesame seeds over the top. Season with salt and pepper and serve.

LEMON VINAIGRETTE

Makes about ⅔ cup

1 large shallot, finely minced

2 tablespoons fresh lemon juice

1 tablespoon rice wine vinegar

Pinch of sea salt

Freshly ground black pepper

⅓ cup extra-virgin olive oil

In a small jar with a lid, combine the shallot, lemon juice, vinegar, and salt. Season with pepper. Let the mixture sit for 15 minutes to soften the shallots, then add the olive oil. Cover and shake vigorously. Store in the refrigerator for up to 4 days. Shake well before using.

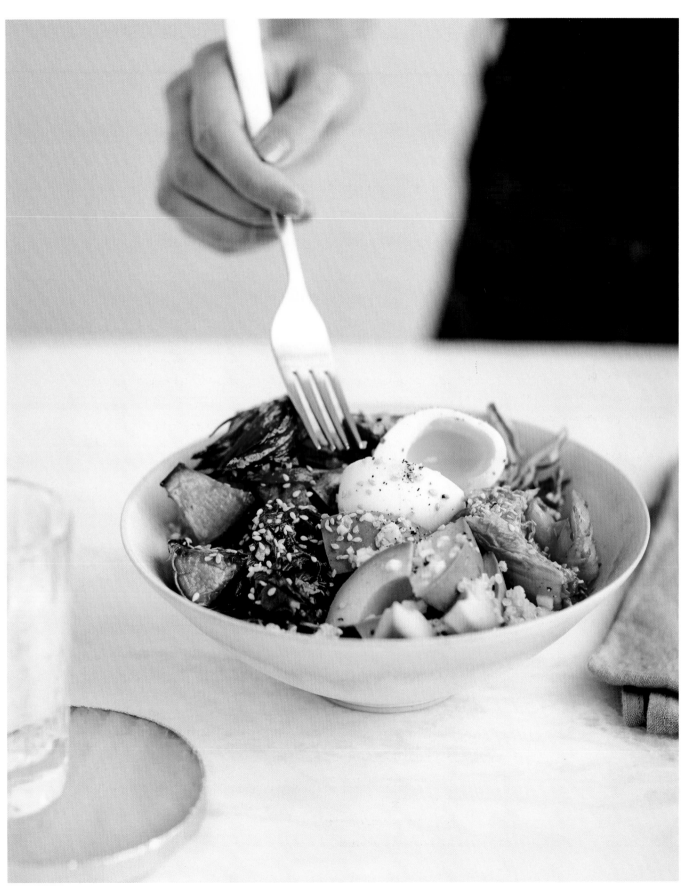

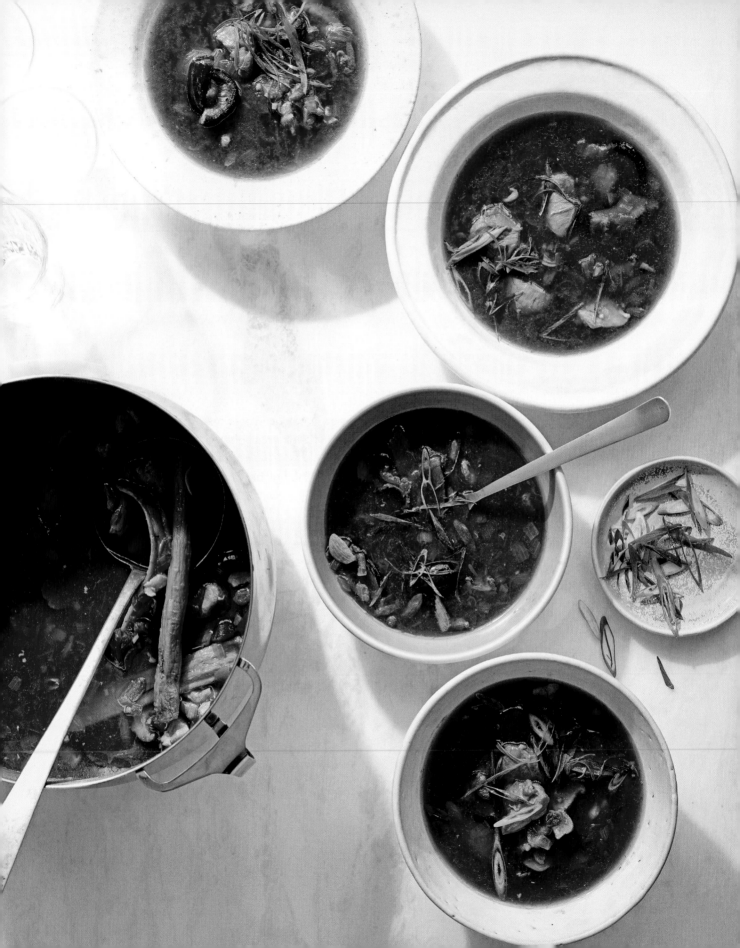

Jill Blakeway, DACM, LAc, a doctor of Traditional Chinese Medicine and acupuncture who's known among New York City women as a fertility guru, developed this delicious immune-boosting chicken soup recipe for another purpose: treating the common cold. (And just dealing with really cold weather in general.) "In Asia the line between food and medicine is more blurred than in the West," says the founder of the Yinova Center. "Chinese medicine is full of recipes that combine food and herbs to make meals that both nourish and cure." You can find these herbs at a Chinese pharmacy, or simmer the broth without them for an equally delicious meal.

HERBAL CHICKEN SOUP

Serves 4

8 da zao (jujubes or red dates), sliced

½ cup gou qi zi (wolfberries)

6 dried shiitake mushrooms, chopped

1 cup boiling water

1 tablespoon olive oil

2 yellow onions, coarsely chopped

Sea salt

6 boneless, skinless chicken thighs, chopped into 1-inch pieces

2 medium red chiles (or to taste), seeded and chopped

1 (2-inch) piece fresh ginger, peeled and finely diced (see Tip, page 226)

4 garlic cloves, thinly sliced

6 cups chicken broth

¼ cup low-sodium soy sauce

3 sticks huang qi (astragalus)

2 (2-inch) pieces dang shen (codonopsis)

1 scallion, sliced

1. In a medium bowl, combine the red dates, wolfberries, and shiitakes. Pour over the boiling water, cover with aluminum foil, and set aside to soak for 20 minutes.

2. Heat the olive oil in a large Dutch oven over medium heat. When it shimmers, add the onions and cook until soft and translucent, about 5 minutes. Season with salt. Increase the heat to medium-high, add the chicken, and cook, stirring, until lightly browned, 5 to 7 minutes. Add the red chiles, ginger, and garlic, and cook, stirring, until fragrant, about 5 minutes more.

3. Pour in the broth and soy sauce, increase the heat to high, and bring to a boil. Reduce the heat to low and simmer gently. Drain the wolfberries, red dates, and shiitakes and add them to the broth with the astragalus and codonopsis. Simmer the soup, with the lid slightly ajar, for 25 to 30 minutes more, until the flavors have melded.

4. Divide the soup among four bowls, garnish with the scallion, and serve.

+

DAIRY-FREE

GLUTEN-FREE

KETOGENIC

LOW-INFLAMMATION

BETTER DIGESTION

BETTER FOCUS

Jenné Claiborne, the voice behind the blog turned cookbook *Sweet Potato Soul*, became a vegan for animal welfare reasons, but quickly realized how veganism also improved her health and happiness. "My food nourishes the body and the soul, and avoids doing harm to the planet and its inhabitants," says the chef, blogger, and cookbook author. This dish is an effortless way for Jenné to showcase her superpower: making delish feel-good food that nourishes the body—and does it quickly! Don't skip soaking the beans the night prior—it takes a little thinking ahead, but makes all the difference.

JENNÉ CLAIBORNE

COCONUT-LIME BLACK BEAN STEW

Serves 4

FOR THE STEW

1 tablespoon coconut oil

1 teaspoon coriander seeds

1 teaspoon cumin seeds

½ red onion, diced

3 garlic cloves, minced

1 tablespoon minced peeled fresh ginger (from one ½-inch piece; see Tip, page 226)

½ yellow bell pepper, diced

1½ cups dried black beans, soaked overnight and drained

1½ cups cubed peeled sweet potato

4 cups vegetable broth

Kosher salt

Cayenne pepper

DAIRY-FREE

GLUTEN-FREE

LOW-INFLAMMATION

VEGAN

VEGETARIAN

BETTER DIGESTION

BETTER FOCUS

FOR THE COCONUT RICE

1½ cups white or brown jasmine rice

¼ teaspoon pink Himalayan salt

1 teaspoon cumin seeds

1 cup full-fat coconut milk (see Tip)

TO ASSEMBLE

1 cup full-fat coconut milk (see Tip)

2 tablespoons fresh lime juice (from about 1 lime)

½ bunch cilantro, for garnish

1 jalapeño, seeded and thinly sliced, for garnish

1. Make the stew. Heat the coconut oil in a large Dutch oven over medium heat. When it shimmers, add the coriander and cumin and fry for about 30 seconds, or until fragrant. Add the onion, garlic, ginger, and bell pepper and cook, stirring, until the onion begins to soften, about 5 minutes. Add the black beans, sweet potato, and broth. Season with salt and cayenne.

2. Increase the heat to high and bring to a boil, then reduce the heat to low and simmer, with the lid ajar, for about 35 minutes, or until the flavors have melded.

3. Meanwhile, make the rice. If using white rice, rinse it in a fine-mesh strainer until the water runs clear. Put the rice in a medium saucepan and add the salt, cumin, and 2½ cups water. Bring to a boil over high heat, then reduce the heat to medium-low. Cook, with the lid ajar, for about 30 minutes, or until the rice is fluffy and the water has been

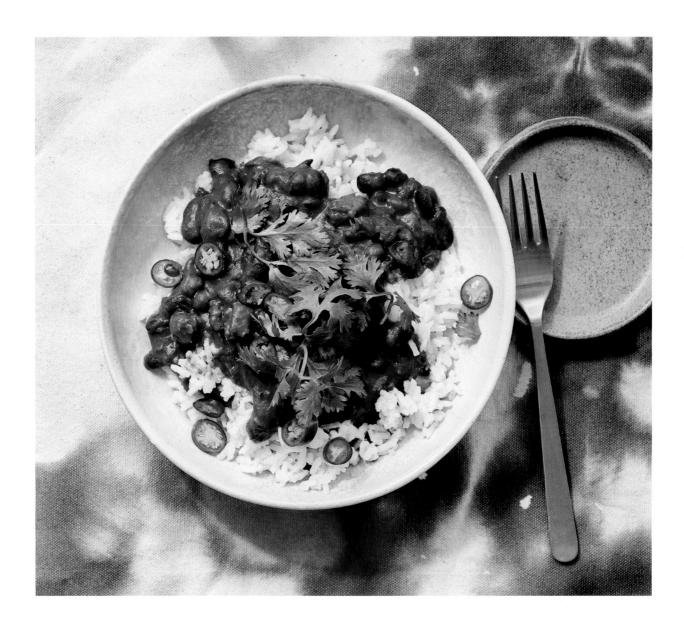

Tip: Between the stew and the rice, you'll be just short on coconut milk if you use a 13.5-ounce can. Make up the difference with water for the rice instead of opening a new can.

absorbed. Stir in the coconut milk and cook for 10 minutes more, or until the liquid has been completely absorbed, adding water as needed if the rice starts to dry out. Fluff the rice with a fork, then cover to keep warm until ready to serve.

4. Finish the stew. When the beans are tender, stir in the coconut milk and lime juice, then cook for 15 to 20 minutes more, until the stew has thickened and the beans are tender. Taste and add more salt and cayenne as needed.

5. Serve the stew over a generous scoop of the coconut rice and garnish with fresh cilantro and jalapeño.

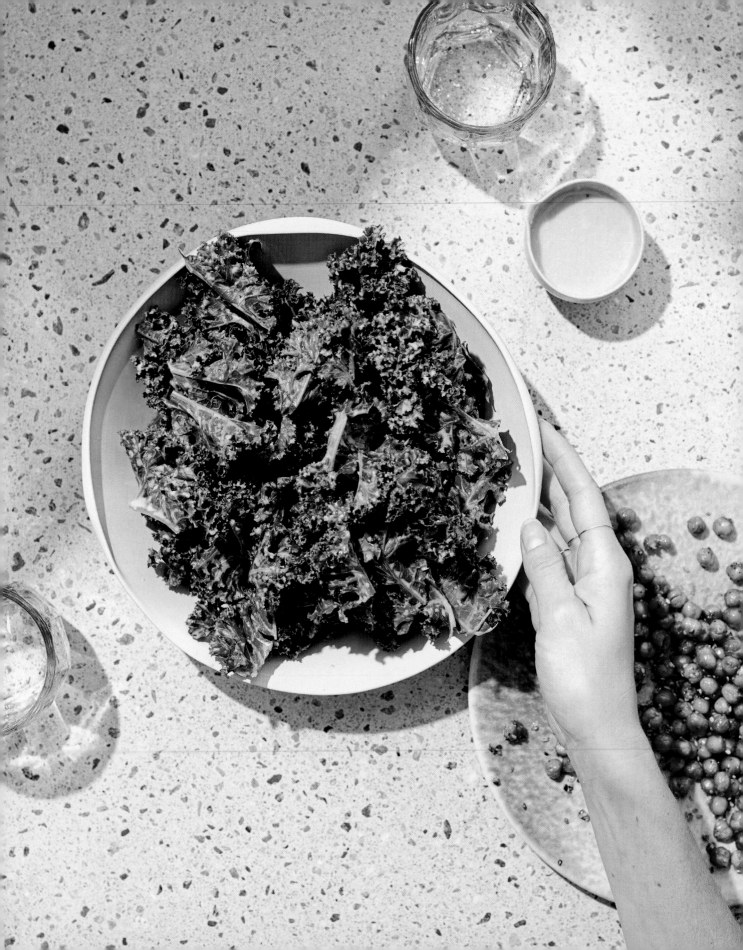

Drew Ramsey, MD, lends his expertise to the Well+Good Council as a Columbia University–based psychiatrist (and farmer!) specializing in exploring the connection between food and brain health. He's also basically the King of Kale, thanks to his cookbook filled with recipes for making the leafy green sexy and focus-forward with boosts of extra-virgin olive oil. This recipe was inspired by the kale growing on his 127-acre organic farm in Indiana—and out of a need for a crunchy crouton substitute. "I'm from the Midwest, so I love a big, traditional dinner—think pasta, pizza, steak— but when I put this salad in my weekly plan, I know I'm winning," he says.

KALE SALAD WITH CHICKPEA CROUTONS

Serves 2 to 4

1 (15-ounce) can chickpeas, drained and rinsed

2 to 3 tablespoons extra-virgin olive oil

¼ teaspoon sea salt, plus more as needed

Freshly ground black pepper, dried oregano, cayenne pepper, and/or smoked paprika (optional)

1 large bunch kale, stemmed, leaves sliced into thin strips or finely chopped

FOR THE DRESSING

2 ounces tinned anchovies, drained

2 garlic cloves

Zest and juice of 1 lemon

2 teaspoons Dijon mustard

2 tablespoons extra-virgin olive oil

¼ cup olive oil–based mayonnaise

1. Preheat the oven to 425°F.

2. Spread the chickpeas in an even layer over a rimmed baking sheet. Add the olive oil, salt, and any additional spices you like, then toss to coat evenly. Roast for 30 to 40 minutes, until crispy.

3. Put the kale in a medium bowl.

4. Make the dressing. In a blender or a food processor, combine the anchovies, garlic, lemon zest, lemon juice, mustard, olive oil, and mayonnaise. Blend until smooth.

5. Add the dressing to the bowl with the kale and toss to coat. Refrigerate until the chickpeas are ready.

6. Remove the chickpeas from the oven and let cool for 1 minute. Sprinkle the chickpeas over the salad, finish with a pinch of salt and a crack of black pepper, and serve immediately.

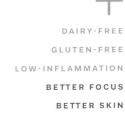

DAIRY-FREE

GLUTEN-FREE

LOW-INFLAMMATION

BETTER FOCUS

BETTER SKIN

Healthy chef Marco Canora couldn't believe how long it took him to discover the perfect hack for polenta: using amaranth instead of stick-to-your-ribs cornmeal mush. "Like other ancient grains, it's packed with an incredible amount of nutrients—one cup of cooked amaranth contains more protein than a hard-boiled egg," says the cookbook author and chef-owner of New York City hotspots Hearth and Brodo, which was an early pioneer of the bone broth trend. Time-saving tip: Marco likes to freeze the kale overnight for easy crumbling instead of wasting precious minutes mincing a fresh bunch.

AMARANTH "POLENTA" WITH TUSCAN KALE

Serves 6

1 bunch Tuscan (lacinato or dinosaur) kale, frozen

6 cups vegetable broth or water

Fine sea salt

2 cups uncooked amaranth

¼ cup freshly grated Parmesan cheese

2 tablespoons extra-virgin olive oil

Freshly ground black pepper

1. Working over a small bowl, crumble the frozen kale leaves with your hands until you have about 1½ cups finely crumbled kale. Discard the stems and thick center ribs.

2. In a large stockpot, combine the broth and 3 big pinches of salt. Bring to a boil over high heat, then reduce the heat to low and, while whisking continuously, pour the amaranth into the water in a slow, steady stream. Stir in the kale and simmer, stirring occasionally, until the mixture reaches a pudding-like consistency, about 30 minutes.

3. Remove the pot from the heat and stir in the cheese, olive oil, and a good dose of pepper. Taste and adjust the seasoning, if needed. Serve hot.

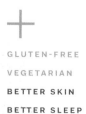

GLUTEN-FREE

VEGETARIAN

BETTER SKIN

BETTER SLEEP

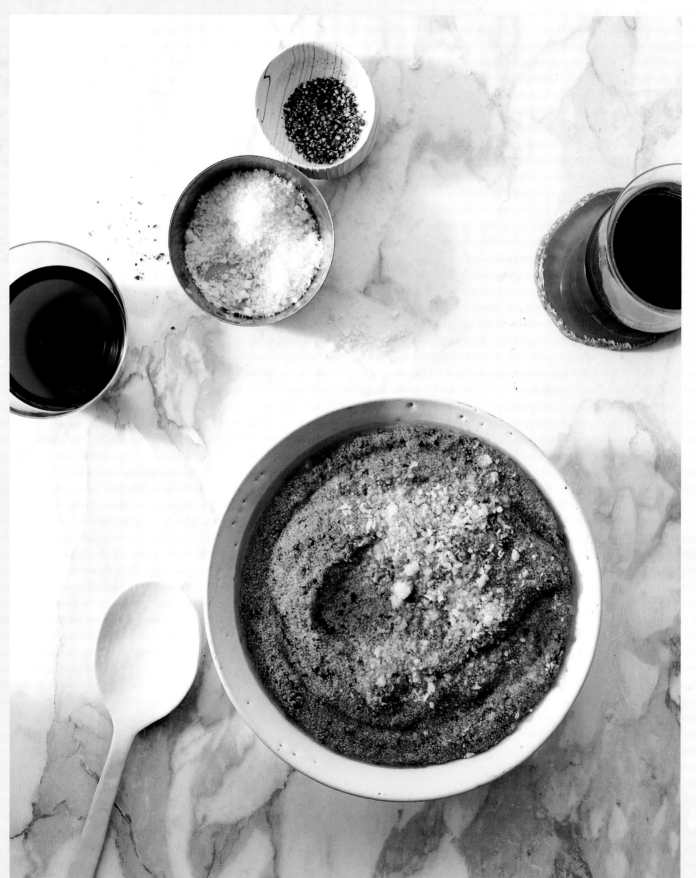

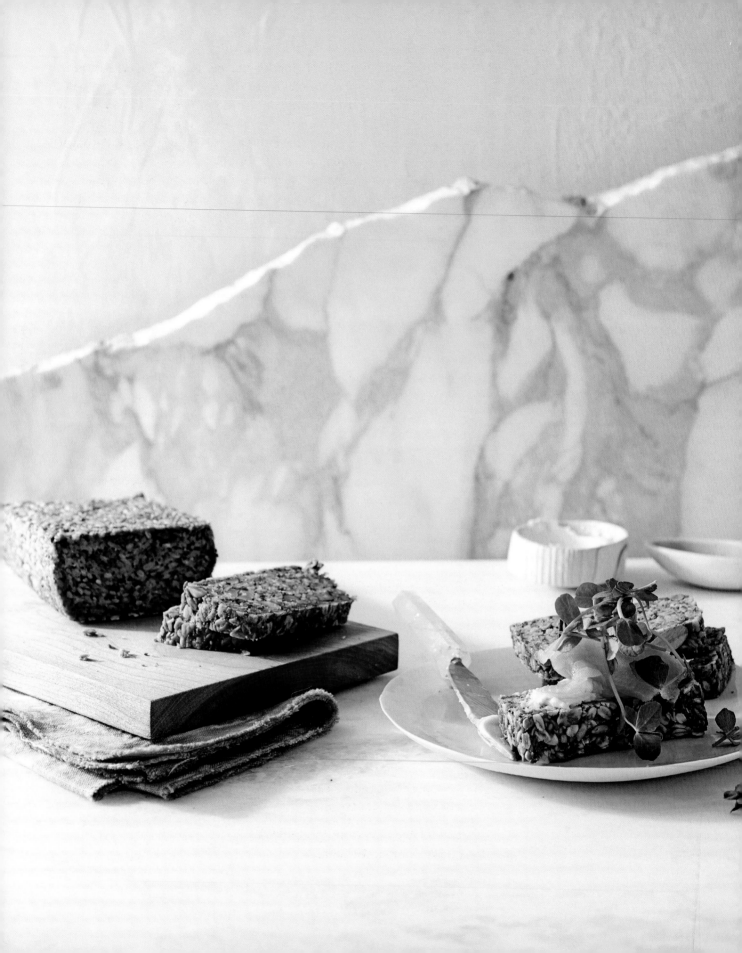

Fashion legend and Well+Good Council member Norma Kamali has the inside scoop—and it has nothing to do with a style trend this time. "Small quantities of simply cooked or raw food with lots of color is the best beauty secret, along with sleep and exercise," says the iconic entrepreneur, who finds inspiration for her fashion collections in wellness, beauty, and women's empowerment. Since gluten isn't on that list, Norma keeps her freezer stocked with this alt-bread for healthy toast (with smoked salmon and tomatoes), an easy lunch (like a hard-boiled egg sandwich with olive oil), or an instant treat (topped with raisins and ginger chunks).

NUT + SEED BREAD

Makes one 12 by 14-inch loaf

1 cup raw sunflower seeds

½ cup flaxseed

½ cup coarsely chopped raw hazelnuts or almonds

1½ cups gluten-free rolled oats

2 tablespoons chia seeds

¼ cup psyllium seed husks, or 3 tablespoons psyllium husk powder

1 teaspoon fine sea salt, or ½ teaspoon coarse sea salt

1 tablespoon pure maple syrup

3 tablespoons coconut oil or ghee, melted

Toppings of your choice

1. In a medium bowl, combine the sunflower seeds, flaxseed, hazelnuts, oats, chia seeds, psyllium, and salt. Mix well with a wooden spoon. In a small bowl, whisk together the maple syrup, melted coconut oil, and 1½ cups water. Add the wet ingredients to the dry ingredients and mix until the dough is well combined and thickened. If the dough is too thick to stir, add 1 to 2 teaspoons more water as needed.

2. Cut a long, thin strip of parchment paper and lay it crosswise in a 12 by 4-inch loaf pan, leaving a 2-inch overhang on both sides. Transfer the mixture to the loaf pan and, using the back of a spoon, smooth out the top. Let the mixture sit in the pan for at least 2 hours or up to 8 hours to ensure the dough retains its shape.

3. About 20 minutes before you're ready to bake the bread, preheat the oven to 350°F.

4. Bake the bread for 20 minutes, then remove it from the oven and, using the overhanging parchment as handles, flip the bread and return it to the pan. Bake for 30 minutes more, or until a tester inserted into the center of the bread comes out clean. Remove from the oven and let the bread cool in the pan for 15 minutes.

5. Turn the bread out of the pan and slice as desired. Top with ingredients of your choosing, such as fresh fruit jam, raisins and ginger chunks, avocado, a hard-boiled egg, or smoked salmon and tomatoes.

6. Store the bread in an airtight container in the freezer for up to 1 month.

+

DAIRY-FREE

GLUTEN-FREE

VEGAN

VEGETARIAN

BETTER DIGESTION

BETTER FOCUS

BETTER SKIN

Chef John Fraser knows his veggies. The mastermind behind Nix—the celebrated plant-based restaurant in New York City—largely sources his ingredients straight from the farmer's market, which inspires fresh menu picks like these tangy dumplings. "The peas contribute a natural sweetness, which the other ingredients play against—the sweet, sour, and umami," says the chef who began his career under the mentorship of Thomas Keller at The French Laundry. Do yourself a favor and fold a bunch of these ahead of time. "Dumplings freeze [basically] forever," says Nix co-owner James Truman. A little prep means you're less than ten minutes away from a Michelin Star–worthy meal.

TOFU-PEA DUMPLINGS

Makes 20 dumplings

¾ cup frozen English peas

¼ (14-ounce) block firm tofu

¼ garlic clove

¼ cup tightly packed fresh mint

⅓ cup olive oil

20 (3½-inch) round dumpling wrappers

TO ASSEMBLE

Chile-Soy Vinaigrette (recipe follows)

Pea sprouts

Snap peas, julienned

Baby heirloom carrots, shaved

1. Fill a large pot (large enough to hold a bamboo steamer or steamer basket) with 2 cups water and bring to a boil over high heat. Line the steamer (or each layer of the bamboo steamer) with a round of parchment paper, but do not put it in the pan yet.

2. In a food processor or a blender, combine the peas, tofu, garlic, mint, and olive oil and pulse until smooth. Make sure to keep the mixture cold, or it will begin to discolor.

3. Place 2 teaspoons of the filling in the center of each dumpling wrapper. Brush the perimeter of the wrapper with a little water. Fold the wrapper in half around the filling (it should look like a half-moon), then brush the ends with a little more water, bring them together, and pinch to seal them.

4. If using a bamboo steamer, place 5 dumplings in each layer; if using a steamer basket, work in batches of 5. Place the steamer in the pot and cook for 5 to 7 minutes, until the dumpling wrappers are opaque. Transfer the cooked dumplings to a plate and repeat to cook the remaining ones.

5. To serve, arrange 5 steamed dumplings in each shallow bowl. Pour over ¼ cup of the vinaigrette. Garnish with sturdy sprouts, julienned snap peas, and shaved baby heirloom carrots, and serve.

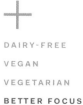

DAIRY-FREE

VEGAN

VEGETARIAN

BETTER FOCUS

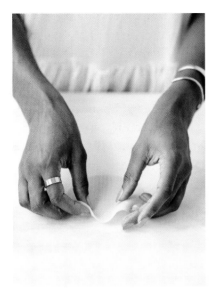

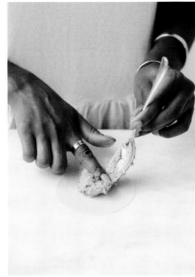

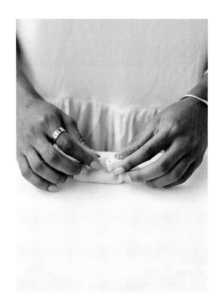

CHILE-SOY VINAIGRETTE

Makes about 1 cup

¾ cup rice wine vinegar

2 tablespoons mirin

¼ cup tamari

1 tablespoon chile oil

In a small bowl, whisk together the vinegar, mirin, tamari, and chile oil until thoroughly combined. Transfer to a squeeze bottle or mason jar with a lid and store in the refrigerator for up to 6 weeks.

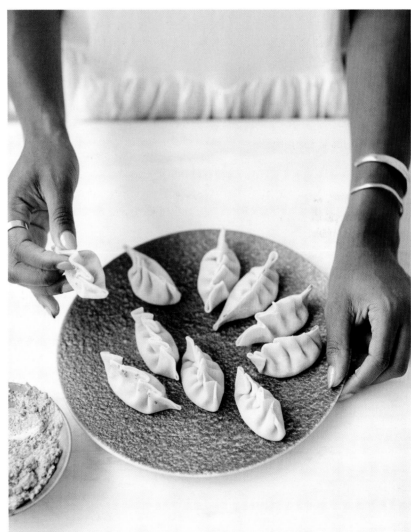

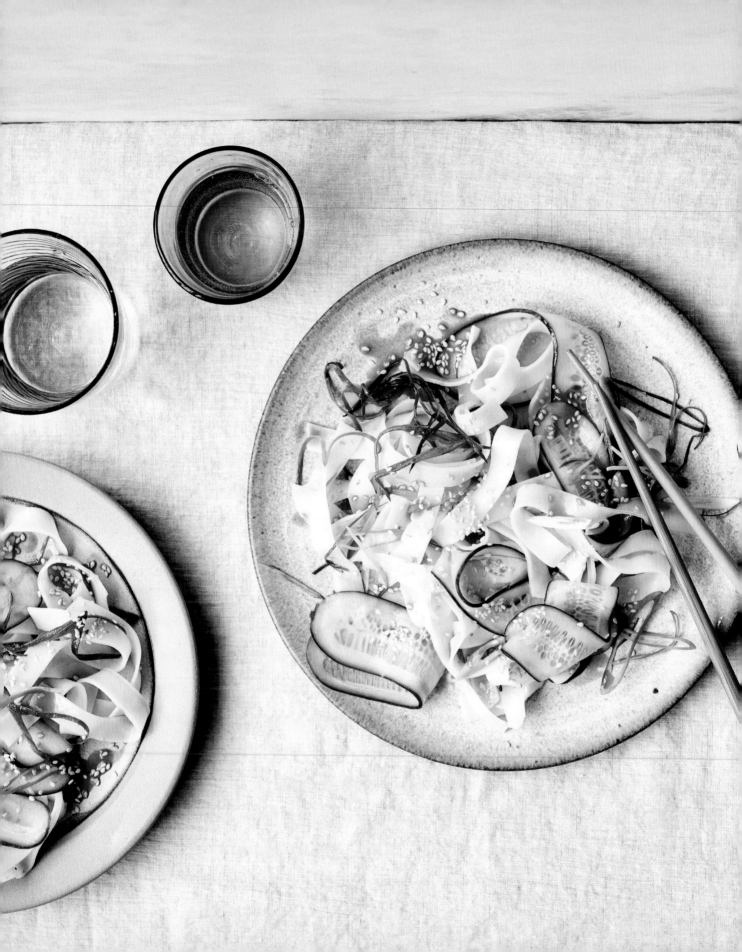

Hot for Food blogger Lauren Toyota admits she can be a little "extra" when it comes to vegan cooking. "I can make an elaborate pasta, no problem," says the author. But with this recipe she embraces her inner minimalist. "I love to make this dish—it's a handful of ingredients that really shine together," she says. While these noodles are relatively no-fuss, Lauren does demand one thing: Get your hands on some high-quality chili oil.

COLD CUCUMBER-CHILI NOODLES

Serves 2

½ pound thick flat rice noodles

1 English cucumber

1 scallion, whites and greens, finely sliced diagonally

1 tablespoon toasted sesame oil

1 tablespoon sesame seeds

⅛ to ¼ teaspoon sea salt

2 tablespoons chili oil

1. Bring a large pot of salted water to a boil over high heat. If your rice noodles already contain salt, do not add salt to the water. Cook the noodles until al dente, about 6 minutes.

2. Meanwhile, cut the cucumber into ribbons using a vegetable peeler or spiralizer, or slice very thinly using a mandolin.

3. Drain the noodles, rinse under cool water, and place in a large bowl. Toss with the cucumber ribbons, scallions, sesame oil, 2 teaspoons of the sesame seeds, and salt to taste.

4. Divide the noodles between the serving plates. Drizzle each serving with ½ tablespoon of chili oil (if you don't like it spicy, use more sesame oil instead) and garnish with the remaining sesame seeds, leaving the cucumber ribbons and scallions to place on top of the noodles.

5. Serve cold or refrigerate in an airtight container for 2 to 3 days.

Tip: Got leftovers? You can soften the noodles by heating them with a bit of water in a covered pan. Drain any excess water before serving.

DAIRY-FREE

GLUTEN-FREE

VEGAN

VEGETARIAN

BETTER SKIN

BETTER SLEEP

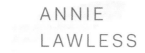
"Every single meal is an opportunity to nourish your body and do something good for yourself," says Annie Lawless, cofounder of the organic cold-pressed juice company Suja Juice, who's now running her own nontoxic beauty brand, Lawless Beauty. When it comes to mealtime, she goes for unprocessed foods that give her body the nutrition it needs, like this *tom kha* soup filled with healthy veggies, spices, and herbs—the ultimate comfort food at the end of a long day.

TOM KHA SOUP WITH SHRIMP

Serves 4

2 tablespoons coconut oil

3 garlic cloves, minced

1 (½-inch) piece fresh ginger, peeled and grated (see Tip, page 226)

1 bunch scallions, thinly sliced

1 medium jalapeño, seeded and minced

2 cups sliced shiitake mushrooms

Sea salt

2½ cups chicken broth

2 (13.5-ounce) cans full-fat coconut milk

2 tablespoons fresh lime juice

2 tablespoons fish sauce (optional)

1 teaspoon sriracha (optional)

Freshly ground black pepper

1 pound fresh medium shrimp, peeled (tails removed) and deveined

¼ cup chopped fresh basil, for garnish

Lime wedges, for serving

1. Melt the coconut oil in a large stockpot over medium heat. Add the garlic, ginger, scallions, jalapeño, and shiitake mushrooms and season with salt. Cook, stirring occasionally, for 5 to 7 minutes, until the vegetables have softened.

2. Add the broth, coconut milk, lime juice, and the fish sauce and sriracha (if using), and season with salt and pepper. Increase the heat to high to bring the mixture to a boil, then reduce the heat to low and simmer for 7 minutes, or until the flavors have melded.

3. Add the shrimp and cook for 3 to 4 minutes, until pink, opaque, and cooked through.

4. Remove the pot from the heat, taste, and season with salt and pepper as needed. Divide the soup among four bowls, garnish with the basil and lime wedges, and serve.

DAIRY-FREE

GLUTEN-FREE

KETOGENIC

LOW-INFLAMMATION

PALEO

BETTER FOCUS

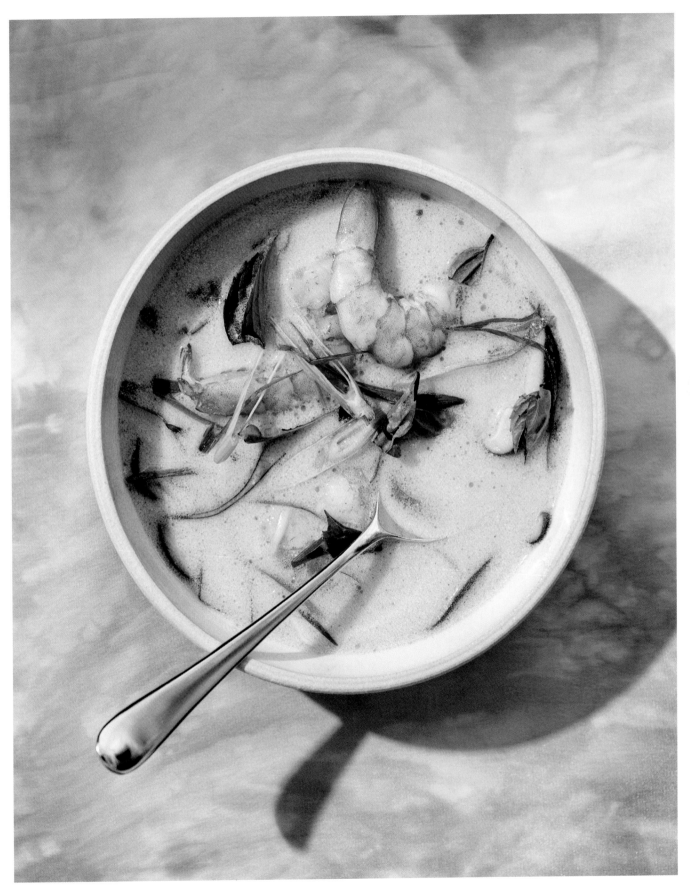

MAINS

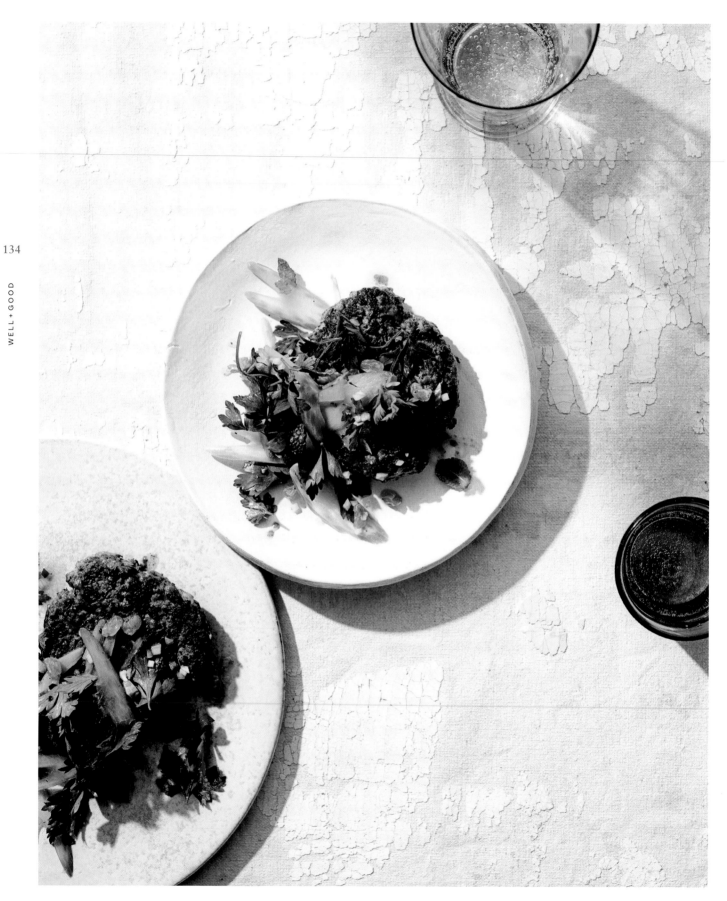

In this dish, Emmy Award–winning television host, author, and chef Daphne Oz combines zucchini and celery for a low-carb, high-fiber main that is extremely hydrating (yes, hydrating!) and excellent for digestion. "The riboflavin in zucchini boosts the health of hair, skin, and nails," says Daphne. What does that mean for you? This vibrant recipe not only packs in the protein, but can also help maintain glowing, plump skin. Timing tip: You'll want to cook these burgers slow enough for the inside to finish cooking before the outside chars.

ZUCCHINI-LAMB BURGERS WITH CELERY SLAW

Makes 4 burgers

FOR THE SLAW

1 tablespoon red wine vinegar

1 small shallot, minced

½ teaspoon dried oregano

Juice of 1 orange

Kosher salt and freshly ground black pepper to taste

¼ cup olive oil

6 celery stalks, thinly sliced, plus ½ cup torn celery leaves

1 cup torn flat leaf parsley leaves, plus minced tender stems

¼ cup torn fresh mint leaves

2 tablespoons golden raisins

FOR THE BURGERS

1 pound ground lamb

2 cups coarsely grated zucchini

6 scallions, thinly sliced

2 tablespoons finely chopped fresh mint leaves

1 teaspoon ground cumin

1 teaspoon kosher salt

Zest of ½ orange

Freshly ground black pepper

2 to 3 tablespoons olive oil

1. Make the slaw. In a medium bowl, whisk together the red wine vinegar, shallot, oregano, juice from the orange, salt, and pepper. Slowly add the olive oil, whisking continuously, until emulsified. Add the celery, parsley, mint, and golden raisins, toss to combine, and set aside.

2. Make the burgers. In a large bowl, combine the lamb, zucchini, scallions, mint, cumin, salt, orange zest, and pepper. With clean hands, gently mix until the zucchini, scallions, and mint are evenly distributed. Wet your hands and divide the mixture into four 1-inch-thick patties.

3. Heat the olive oil in a medium nonstick skillet over medium heat. When it shimmers, add the burger patties, taking care not to overcrowd the pan and working in batches as necessary. Cook for 5 to 6 minutes, then flip and cook for 5 minutes on the second side for medium-well.

4. Remove the burgers from the pan and set aside for 3 to 4 minutes. Top each with a heaping spoonful of slaw and serve.

+

DAIRY-FREE

LOW-INFLAMMATION

PALEO

BETTER SKIN

"My appreciation for and connection to food comes directly from nature," says Michael Lim, executive chef and co-owner of Chikarashi, a poke restaurant in New York City. This Japanese Chinese take on a Hawaiian poke bowl comes from his knowledge of Asian cuisine and his love of pickled vegetables. Here Michael also introduces you to your new best friend, furikake—aka umami seaweed sprinkles—which, along with the bonito flakes and pickled daikon, can be purchased online, at a Japanese grocer, or often in the spice aisle at a regular supermarket. If you don't know, now you know.

SPICY SALMON POKE

Serves 2

¼ cup kosher salt, plus more as needed

2 tablespoons monk fruit sweetener

8 ounces wild salmon fillet, cut into ½-inch cubes

1 small white onion, thinly sliced

2 tablespoons spicy mayonnaise, store-bought or homemade

1 tablespoon olive oil

¼ cup bonito flakes, crumbled

3 cups cooked short-grain sushi rice

2 tablespoons furikake

1 (1-inch) piece pickled daikon, thinly sliced

1 scallion, thinly sliced

1. In a medium bowl, stir together the kosher salt and monk fruit sweetener. Add the salmon and toss to coat completely. Cover and refrigerate for at least 3 hours or up to 12 hours.

2. Rinse the salmon and pat dry. In a clean medium bowl, toss the salmon, onion, and spicy mayo to coat. Season with salt.

3. Heat the olive oil in a small skillet over medium-high heat. When it shimmers, add the bonito flakes and cook, stirring, until toasted, 3 to 4 minutes. Remove the skillet from the heat.

4. Divide the rice between two bowls and sprinkle each with half of the furikake. Add the salmon mixture, pickled daikon, and scallions, dividing them evenly. Sprinkle the toasted bonito flakes over the top and serve immediately.

GLUTEN-FREE

LOW-INFLAMMATION

BETTER DIGESTION

BETTER ENERGY

BETTER FOCUS

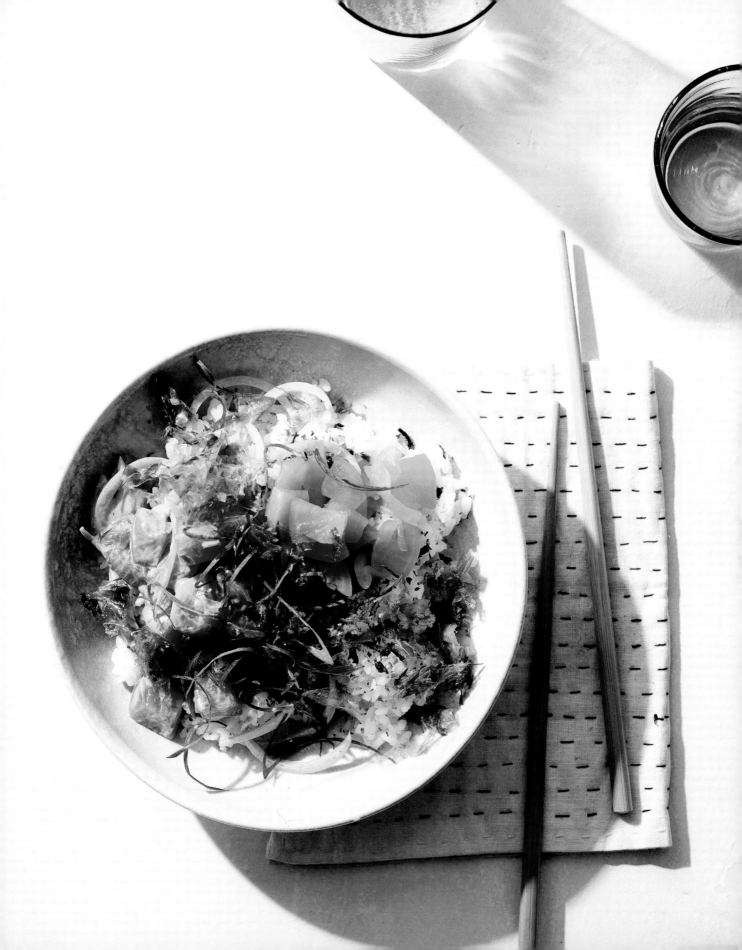

EAT FOR BETTER FOCUS

Because I'm a psychiatrist who also grows crops on my 127-acre Indiana farm, my food approach is basically "farmer meets pharma." Brain molecules are my business, and improving brain health and mental health is how I help people heal. So when we talk about eating for focus, it's really eating for brain health—because focus is a brain phenomenon. And you can change so much with your diet.

> CONSUMING LOTS OF LEAFY GREENS, CRUCIFEROUS AND COLORFUL VEGGIES, AND SENSIBLE SEAFOOD IS KEY TO MAINTAINING FOCUS.

Remember the last time you were "in the zone"? Well, what turns that on? In the brain, focus is most regulated by a chemical called dopamine. Every stimulant, from dark chocolate and matcha to Adderall and Ritalin, works by triggering the release of dopamine. You know that slightly energized, optimistic, time-to-get-stuff-done moment after your first cup of coffee? That's dopamine.

On the other hand, depression zaps focus. And since how you eat is directly related to your risk of depression, consuming lots of leafy greens, cruciferous and colorful veggies, and sensible seafood is key to maintaining focus. And nothing interrupts focus and creativity like anxiety.

Avoiding simple sugars and eating more foods like eggs, which are high in choline (an amino acid), can help with excessive worry.

To help you dial in your meal plan for laser-like focus, make sure your pantry is stocked with these foods:

EXTRA-VIRGIN OLIVE OIL. Use EVOO generously. Good fats are good for your brain health. Use it in your cooking, and keep a small bottle at work to make salad dressing with a squeeze of lemon juice. (Bottled salad dressings are usually filled with low-quality oils, artificial flavors, and added sugar.)

CASHEWS. Cashews are high in magnesium, iron, and zinc—three minerals that are key for focus.

FISH. Salmon and tuna are great, but smaller oily fish like anchovies and sardines that are rich in omega-3 fatty acids are the unsung heroes of brain foods. Adding them to a salad or salad dressing tones down their fishiness a bit. Once you're acclimatized to their salty flavor, they make a great snack on a rice cake.

DARK CHOCOLATE. Dark chocolate contains healthy flavonoids that some science shows improve memory and protect brain cells. It is also high in fiber, iron, and magnesium.

—DREW RAMSEY, MD

"My whole life, I've been fortunate to have a positive, happy relationship with food," says Lea Michele, the actress, singer, and author. "Food always meant family, it meant laughter, it meant happiness." Growing up, Lea remembers sitting down for Sunday dinners with her Italian family, but only as she got older did she learn the importance of food as fuel. In this recipe, she gives (mostly) homemade pizza a boost with high-fiber radicchio, upping its make-your-own party potential with better-for-digestion ingredients. Choose a crust, from wheat to cauliflower, to personalize your pie.

SHAVED RADICCHIO, PARMESAN + TRUFFLE PIZZA

Makes one 12-inch pizza

1 medium head radicchio, finely shaved (about 1½ cups)

Juice of 1 lemon

1 teaspoon kosher salt

2 tablespoons plus 1 teaspoon olive oil, plus more for drizzling

1 premade 12-inch pizza crust (may be gluten-free), cooked

½ cup freshly shaved Parmesan cheese

Freshly ground black pepper (optional)

1 large egg

1 teaspoon truffle oil (optional)

Crushed red pepper flakes (optional)

1. Preheat the oven to 425°F.

2. In a medium bowl, combine the radicchio, lemon juice, kosher salt, and 2 tablespoons of the olive oil. Toss to coat the radicchio.

3. Place the pizza crust on a baking sheet, then layer the radicchio on top of the crust, leaving a 1-inch border. Drizzle a bit of olive oil over the top and bake until the radicchio is crispy, about 10 minutes.

4. Remove the pizza from the oven and sprinkle the Parmesan over the whole surface. Add a few cracks of black pepper, if desired, and bake for 3 minutes more, or until the cheese has melted.

5. Meanwhile, heat the remaining 1 teaspoon olive oil in a small skillet over medium heat. When it shimmers, crack the egg into the pan. Reduce the heat to low and cook until the egg white is completely set but the yolk is still runny, about 3 minutes. Use a spatula to slide the sunny-side-up egg on top of the pizza and bake for 2 minutes more (or turn on the broiler and broil to make the pizza extra crispy).

6. Before serving, drizzle with the truffle oil and sprinkle with red pepper flakes, if desired.

GLUTEN-FREE

VEGETARIAN

BETTER DIGESTION

BETTER FOCUS

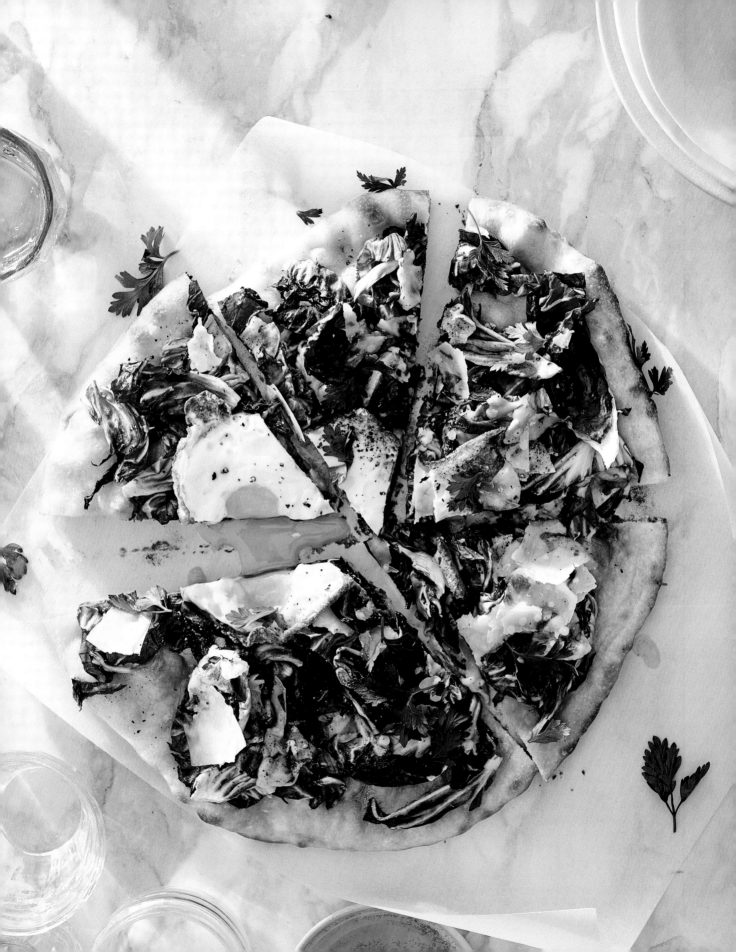

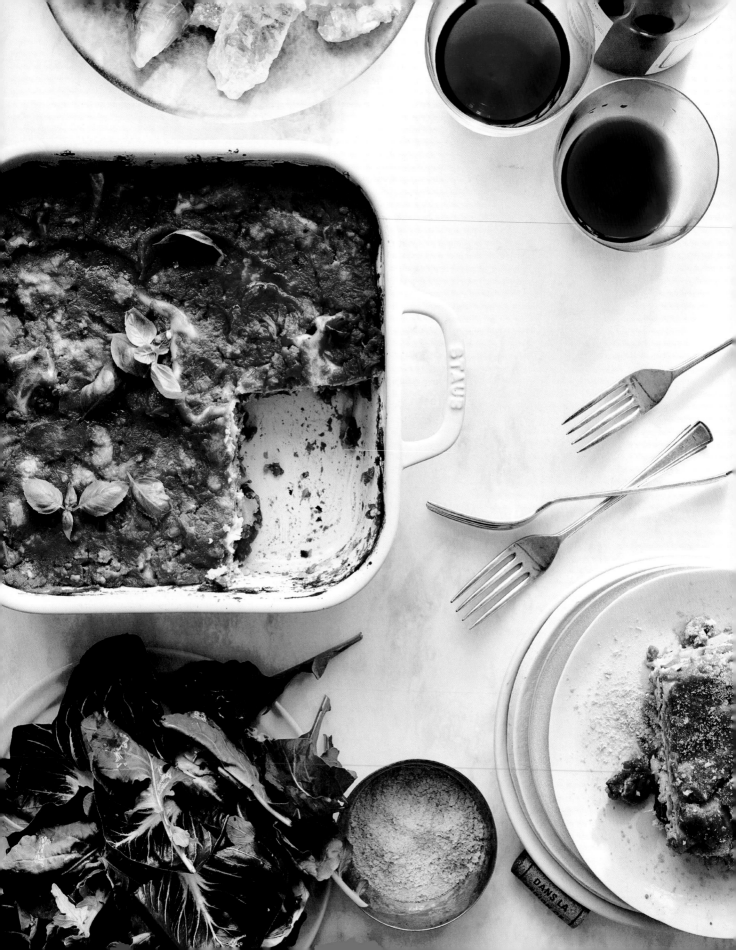

LO
BOSWORTH

"I approach cooking and eating from two perspectives: that food is fuel, and that it should be delicious," says Lo Bosworth, the wellness entrepreneur who runs a lifestyle site, TheLoDown, as well as Love Wellness, a line of better-for-you feminine-care products. In this gluten- and dairy-free dish, Lo uses spices and fresh herbs to infuse delicious flavor while giving the Italian classic a makeover with brain-boosting cashew cheese. "There's no reason healthy foods have to be boring or unappealing," she says. Lean on a few fresh herbs instead. Pro tip: Don't exceed low heat while cooking the turkey, or the meat will lose moisture.

CASHEW-RICOTTA TURKEY LASAGNA

Serves 4

FOR THE CASHEW CHEESE

1½ cups raw cashews, soaked in hot water for at least 1 hour or up to overnight and drained

1 tablespoon apple cider vinegar

2 tablespoons nutritional yeast

Pinch of sea salt

FOR THE LASAGNA

2 tablespoons extra-virgin olive oil

3 garlic cloves, minced

½ yellow onion, diced

Kosher salt

1 pound 90% lean ground turkey

Freshly ground black pepper

7 cups diced peeled tomatoes (from three 28-ounce cans, drained)

1 teaspoon dried oregano

1½ cups chopped fresh basil

About 20 oven-ready gluten-free lasagna noodles (from about two 9-ounce packages)

1 cup spinach

Nutritional yeast (optional)

1. Preheat the oven to 375°F.

2. Make the cashew cheese. In a food processor, pulse the cashews briefly just to break them a bit, then add the vinegar, nutritional yeast, salt, and ½ cup water and pulse until the mixture has a fluffy, ricotta-like consistency.

3. Make the lasagna. Heat the olive oil in a large skillet over medium heat. When it shimmers, add the garlic and cook, stirring, for 30 seconds, or until fragrant. Add the onion and a pinch of salt, reduce the heat to medium-low, and cook, stirring often, for 5 minutes, or until the onion is soft and translucent.

4. Reduce the heat to low. Add the ground turkey, season generously with salt and pepper, and cook, breaking up the meat with a wooden spoon as it cooks, until the turkey is about halfway done, with some areas still pink, about 5 to 7 minutes. Add the tomatoes, oregano, and basil, increase the heat to medium, and bring to a simmer. Season with salt and pepper and cook for about 30 minutes to allow the flavors to come together.

5. Spread one-quarter of the sauce over the bottom of a 9-inch square baking dish, then add a layer of lasagna noodles, overlapping them as needed. Add one-third of the remaining sauce, followed by ¼ cup of the spinach, then ¼ cup of the cashew cheese. Repeat the layers three or four more times: noodles, sauce, spinach, cheese, with the final layer omitting the spinach. Sprinkle extra basil and additional nutritional yeast on top, if desired.

6. Bake for 30 to 35 minutes, until the lasagna is bubbling and cooked through. Let cool slightly, then slice into squares and serve warm.

DAIRY-FREE

GLUTEN-FREE

BETTER FOCUS

BETTER SLEEP

"My food philosophy centers around vibrant, colorful food that fuels and nourishes, keeping you healthy so you can take on the world," says Dan Churchill, the cookbook author, healthy chef at Under Armour, and cofounder of the Aussie-inspired New York City restaurant Charley St. "My mission is super simple: to use food as a tool to bring people together and enrich their daily lives." He came up with this recipe out of his love for cooking for friends—because what's better than the sweet potato, both as a vitamin-rich dish *and* a crowd-pleaser? Dan likes to serve this gnocchi simply, but you can also caramelize them in olive oil before topping with your favorite pasta sauce.

SWEET POTATO GNOCCHI

Serves 2 to 4

Kosher salt

2 large sweet potatoes

1 large egg, beaten

1 cup oat flour, gluten-free flour, or all-purpose flour, plus more as needed

Kosher salt and freshly ground black pepper

Olive oil, for serving

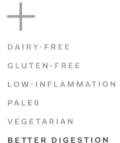

DAIRY-FREE

GLUTEN-FREE

LOW-INFLAMMATION

PALEO

VEGETARIAN

BETTER DIGESTION

BETTER ENERGY

1. Preheat the oven to 425°F.

2. Sprinkle some kosher salt onto a large baking sheet. Prick the sweet potatoes all over with a fork and put them on the pan. Bake for 30 to 40 minutes, until soft. Remove from the oven and let the potatoes cool slightly. When they are cool enough to handle, separate the flesh from the skins (don't worry if it crumbles a bit), discarding the skins. Return the flesh to the baking sheet to dry out, about 20 minutes.

3. Bring a large pot of water to a boil over high heat. Salt the water.

4. Transfer the sweet potato flesh to a medium bowl and add the egg, oat flour, and a pinch each of kosher salt and pepper. Using a spatula, mix until the ingredients are evenly combined and smooth.

5. Test the dough by using your palms to roll a thumbnail-size piece into a ball. Drop the ball into the boiling water and cook for 4 to 5 minutes, until it rises to the top. If it falls apart in the water, discard it and add a pinch more oat flour to the dough. Test again using the same process. If the dough stays firmly together, form the gnocchi.

6. On a floured surface, roll the dough into thin logs, then cut the logs crosswise into thumbnail-size pieces.

7. Working in batches as needed to avoid overcrowding, drop the gnocchi into the boiling water and cook for 4 to 5 minutes, until they rise to the top.

8. Drain the gnocchi in a colander and let cool slightly.

9. Divide the gnocchi among two to four bowls. Drizzle with olive oil, sprinkle with salt, and serve.

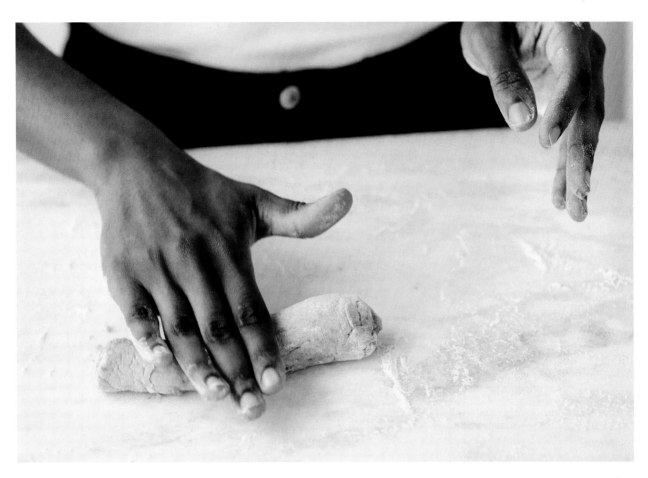

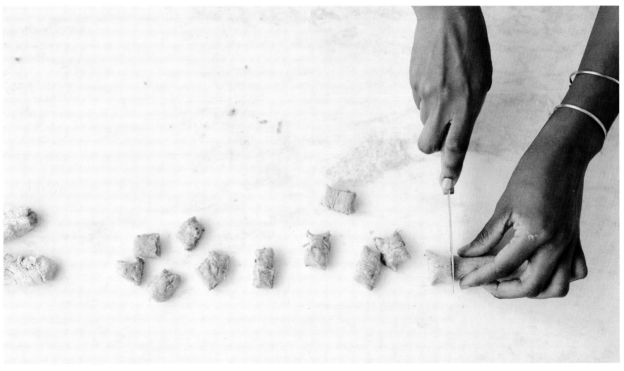

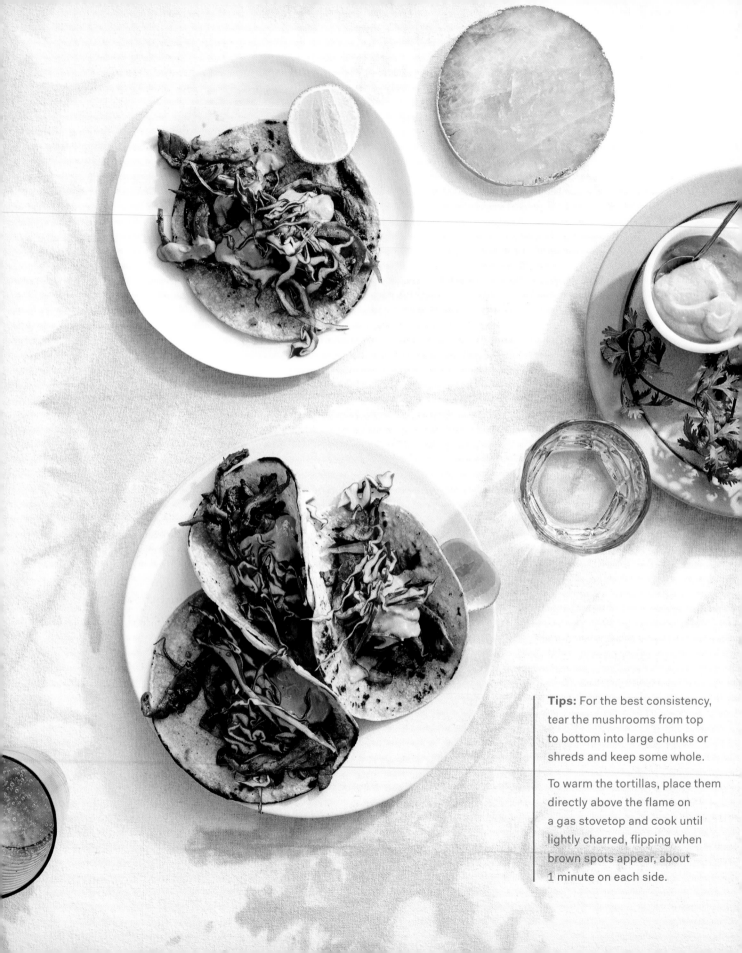

Tips: For the best consistency, tear the mushrooms from top to bottom into large chunks or shreds and keep some whole.

To warm the tortillas, place them directly above the flame on a gas stovetop and cook until lightly charred, flipping when brown spots appear, about 1 minute on each side.

WHITNEY
TINGLE
+
DANIELLE
DUBOISE

"Food should make you feel sexy," say Whitney Tingle and Danielle DuBoise, founders of Sakara Life, an organic, plant-based meal delivery and wellness brand. While avocado is known as a libido booster (thanks, vitamin B_6), Whitney and Danielle are also all about this recipe for its pro-immunity antioxidants, brain-friendly fats, and metabolism-revving spices. The oyster mushrooms, coated with homemade savory seasoning, bring the heat. Make this when you need to spice up your weeknight.

PULLED MUSHROOM TACOS
WITH AVOCADO-LIME TAHINI

Serves 3 or 4

FOR THE SAUCE

1 avocado, pitted and peeled

½ cup fresh cilantro

2 garlic cloves

2 tablespoons tahini

Juice of 2 limes (about ¼ cup)

1 small jalapeño, seeded and diced

½ cup filtered water, plus more as needed

Sea salt and black pepper

FOR THE TACOS

1½ to 3 teaspoons chili powder

¼ teaspoon garlic powder

¼ teaspoon onion powder

¼ teaspoon red pepper flakes

¼ teaspoon dried oregano

½ teaspoon paprika

1 teaspoon ground cumin

1 teaspoon sea salt

1 tablespoon avocado oil

1 small shallot, diced

6 cups oyster mushrooms, torn (see Tip)

TO ASSEMBLE

Warmed corn tortillas (see Tip) or whole Bibb lettuce leaves, for serving

3 cups shredded purple cabbage (from about 1 small or ½ large head)

Lime wedges, for serving

1. Make the sauce. In a blender or food processor, combine the avocado, cilantro, garlic, tahini, lime juice, jalapeño, and filtered water and season with salt and black pepper. Blend until completely smooth, adding more filtered water as needed. Refrigerate until ready to use.

2. Make the tacos. In a small bowl, stir together the chili powder (using more or less to taste), garlic powder, onion powder, red pepper flakes, oregano, paprika, cumin, and salt until evenly combined.

3. Heat the avocado oil in a large skillet over medium heat. When it shimmers, add the shallot and cook, stirring, until soft and translucent, about 3 minutes. Stir in the mushrooms, then add the taco seasoning. Cook, stirring, until the mushrooms begin to soften, 6 to 8 minutes.

4. To assemble, divide the mushroom filling among the warm tortillas. Top each with some shredded cabbage and the sauce. Serve with lime wedges alongside for squeezing.

+

DAIRY-FREE

GLUTEN-FREE

LOW-INFLAMMATION

VEGAN

VEGETARIAN

BETTER SEX

BETTER SKIN

This recipe is a sentimental favorite for ballerina extraordinaire Misty Copeland. "It's the first dish I taught my husband, Olu Evans, how to make," says the prestigious American Ballet Theatre's first African American female principal dancer. Misty loves collards, but considering that they take a long time to cook, she swaps in kale for her busy weeknight greens. Not only does it get this delicious dish on the table faster, the nutrient-rich leafy greens help keep energy levels high for peak performance.

SAUTÉED FLOUNDER WITH KALE

Serves 2

FOR THE KALE

2 tablespoons extra-virgin olive oil

1 small yellow onion, diced

Sea salt

1 tablespoon crushed red pepper flakes, or to taste

4 garlic cloves, minced

2 small bunches kale, stemmed

2 cups low-sodium vegetable broth

Splash of white wine vinegar

Freshly ground black pepper

FOR THE FLOUNDER

2 tablespoons extra-virgin olive oil

6 ounces flounder

Kosher salt and freshly ground black pepper

Hot sauce, for serving

DAIRY-FREE

GLUTEN-FREE

KETOGENIC

LOW-INFLAMMATION

PALEO

BETTER ENERGY

BETTER FOCUS

BETTER SKIN

1. Make the kale. Heat the olive oil in a large pot over high heat. When it shimmers, add the onion and season with salt. Reduce the heat to medium-low and cook for 3 to 4 minutes, until the onion is soft and translucent. Add the red pepper flakes and garlic. Cook, stirring, for about 1 minute, or until fragrant.

2. Add the kale. Pour in the broth, increase the heat to high, and bring the broth to a boil. Add the vinegar and season with salt and black pepper. Reduce the heat to low and simmer for 25 minutes, or until the kale is completely wilted.

3. Meanwhile, make the flounder. Heat the olive oil in a medium nonstick skillet over medium-high heat. Season the flounder all over with salt and black pepper. When the oil shimmers, add the fish skin-side up. Cook until golden brown on the bottom, about 3 minutes, then flip the fish over and cook for 2 to 3 minutes more, until no longer translucent.

4. Divide the kale between two plates and season with hot sauce. Place the flounder on top and serve immediately.

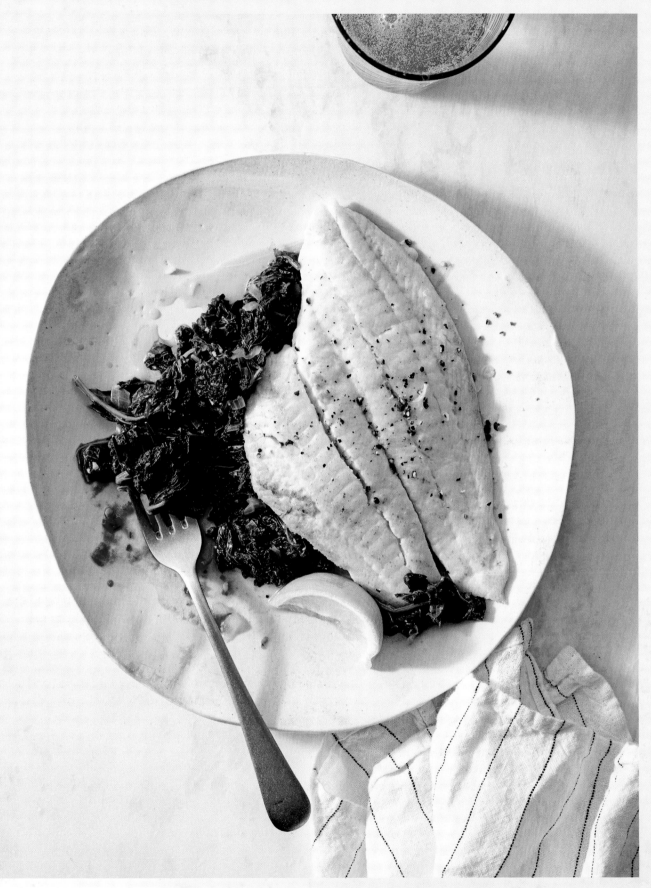

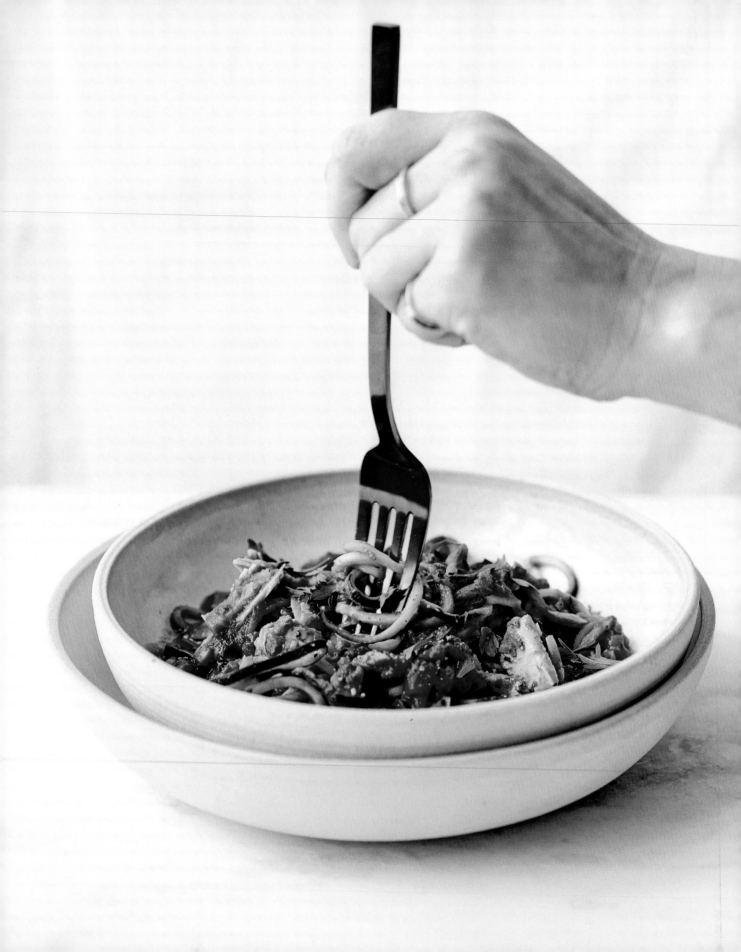

BOBBI
BROWN

"Health and wellness are not new concepts for me," says beauty boss Bobbi Brown. "I have always believed that the better you take care of yourself on the inside, the better you look on the outside." With a cosmetics empire built (and sold) on a radiant, natural look and a new wellness company, Evolution_18, Bobbi is serious about skin—and this veggie-packed recipe is one of her favorites for inside-out gorgeousness. The quick-sauté dish can be doubled (or quadrupled!) to feed multiple people—and vegans and Meatless Monday advocates can sub in cannellini beans for the canned tuna without losing any Italian-spiced flavor.

SPIRALIZED ZUCCHINI PASTA
WITH ITALIAN SPICES + TUNA

Serves 1

1 teaspoon olive oil

1 teaspoon thinly sliced garlic

1 teaspoon dried parsley

1 teaspoon chopped sun-dried tomato

1 teaspoon crushed red pepper flakes

1 large zucchini, spiralized (about 2 cups)

1 (5-ounce) can Italian tuna packed in oil, drained

1½ cups prepared marinara sauce

Kosher salt and freshly ground black pepper

1 tablespoon chopped fresh parsley, for serving (optional)

1 tablespoon lemon zest, for serving (optional)

1. Heat the olive oil in a large pan over medium-high heat. When it shimmers, add the garlic, parsley, sun-dried tomato, and red pepper flakes and cook, stirring, until fragrant, 1 to 2 minutes. Add the zucchini and cook until tender but still al dente, with a bit of crunch. Add the tuna and toss to combine.

2. Season the marinara sauce with salt and black pepper and add it to the pan, using a wooden spoon to stir and coat everything evenly with the sauce. Cook for 1 minute, just to warm the sauce through.

3. Transfer to a bowl, top with the parsley and lemon zest, if desired, and serve.

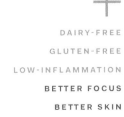

DAIRY-FREE

GLUTEN-FREE

LOW-INFLAMMATION

BETTER FOCUS

BETTER SKIN

Seamus Mullen wasn't always the wellness expert he is today. After a brain infection landed him in the ER with a fever close to 106°F, the chef was forced to rethink his relationship with food, and he ultimately removed refined sugar, dairy, and gluten from his kitchen to combat his rheumatoid arthritis. He now sticks closely to a Paleo diet. "I'm a big advocate of balance within a dish," says Seamus. "That means giving an equally important role to vegetables as to protein—and balancing the phunk: sweet and spicy, salty and sour." We vote you steal Seamus's matcha cashew trick for your new signature kitchen hack and bottle his tangy vinaigrette for dressing greens on the go.

PHUNKY CHICKEN SALAD
WITH MATCHA CASHEWS

Serves 4

FOR THE VINAIGRETTE

¼ cup fresh lime juice
(from about 2 limes)

¼ cup fresh lemon juice
(from 1 or 2 lemons)

2 tablespoons rice wine vinegar

3 tablespoons coconut oil,
melted

3 tablespoons olive oil

2 tablespoons yuzu juice

Sea salt

GLUTEN-FREE

LOW-INFLAMMATION

PALEO

BETTER FOCUS

BETTER SKIN

FOR THE SLAW

¼ head red cabbage, sliced
(about 2 cups)

¼ head napa cabbage, sliced
(about 2 cups)

½ cup pickled carrots

Fish sauce (optional)

Sea salt

FOR THE SALAD

½ cup raw cashews

1 tablespoon matcha green tea powder

1 teaspoon sea salt, plus more
as needed

2 cups arugula

Leaves from 3 sprigs basil, torn

Leaves from 3 sprigs cilantro, torn

Leaves from 2 sprigs mint, torn

1 cup julienned pear

1 cup shredded rotisserie chicken meat

½ large English cucumber, quartered
lengthwise and thinly sliced

1 cup pickled jalapeños

2 cups cauliflower rice
(or see Tip on page 62)

1. Make the vinaigrette. In a small bowl, whisk together the lime juice, lemon juice, vinegar, melted coconut oil, olive oil, and yuzu juice. Season with salt.

2. Make the slaw. In a medium bowl, combine the red cabbage, napa cabbage, pickled carrots, vinaigrette to taste, and fish sauce (if using). Season with salt and toss to combine thoroughly. Set aside.

3. Make the salad. In a food processor, combine the cashews, matcha, and salt and pulse just until the nuts are coated and crumbly.

4. In a large serving bowl, combine the arugula, basil, cilantro, mint, pear, chicken, cucumber, jalapeños, cauliflower rice, matcha cashews, and cabbage slaw. Season with salt. Add ⅓ cup of the vinaigrette and toss to coat well and combine evenly. Serve immediately.

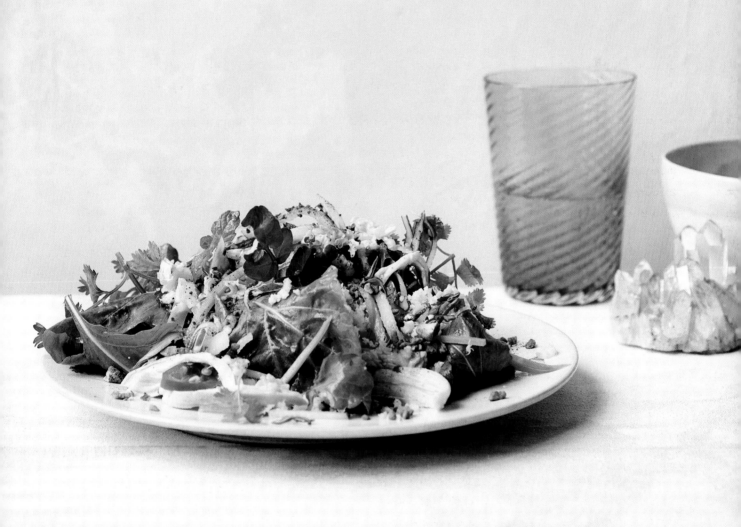

Tip: Adding turmeric to your poaching water will dye the eggs yellow for a natural pop of color in the dish.

Gabe Kennedy believes that food is a "gateway to culture, tradition, people, and history"—something the globe-trotting, often-televised chef has learned from experience. "Food holds enormous power," he says. Gabe, who's also cofounder of Plant People, a wellness brand that creates CBD foods and supplements, often finds himself making this recipe when his fridge is not so well-stocked, whether before or after jetting off on a culinary adventure. The yolk acts as a makeshift sauce, coating the focus-enhancing lentils and mood-boosting chard.

WARMED LENTILS WITH POACHED EGG

Serves 2

FOR THE LENTILS

3 tablespoons olive oil

1 tablespoon minced peeled fresh ginger (from about one ½-inch piece)

2 garlic cloves, minced

1 small white onion, finely chopped

⅓ teaspoon ground coriander

1 teaspoon ground turmeric

¼ teaspoon black pepper

Pink Himalayan salt

3 cups vegetable broth

1 cup beluga lentils

FOR THE EGGS

4 large eggs

2 tablespoons distilled white vinegar

Pinch of ground turmeric (optional)

TO ASSEMBLE

1 teaspoon sherry vinegar

¼ cup currants

3 cups torn Swiss chard leaves

Pink Himalayan salt and black pepper

Flaky sea salt, olive oil, mint, and cilantro

1. Make the lentils. Heat the olive oil in a medium saucepan over medium heat. When it shimmers, add the ginger, garlic, onion, coriander, turmeric, and pepper. Season with salt. Cook, stirring, until the vegetables are soft and fragrant, about 5 minutes, taking care not to burn the spices. Add the broth and the lentils and increase to high heat to bring the broth to a boil. Reduce the heat to low, cover, and simmer until the lentils are tender, 30 to 40 minutes.

2. Meanwhile, poach the eggs. Fill a small saucepan with 4 inches of water and bring to a boil over high heat. One at a time, crack each egg into a small bowl or ramekin. Add the white vinegar and turmeric (if using) to the water. Gently stirring the water to create a vortex, slide an egg into the center.

3. While continuing to stir to maintain the vortex, cook the egg for 3 to 4 minutes, until the whites are set but the yolk is still runny. Gently remove with a slotted spoon and place it on a clean kitchen towel to drain. Repeat with the remaining eggs.

4. To assemble, add the sherry vinegar, currants, and chard to the lentils and stir to combine. Season with salt and pepper.

5. Divide the lentils among two bowls and top each with two poached eggs, some flaky salt, olive oil, and fresh herbs.

GLUTEN-FREE

KETOGENIC

LOW-INFLAMMATION

PALEO

VEGETARIAN

BETTER FOCUS

BETTER MOOD

"Health starts in the kitchen," says writer My Nguyen, who created the blog *My Healthy Dish* based on the goings-on in her own kitchen. All the recipes she shares on her popular Instagram account are first made at home for her family—and this pho shows up on her dinner table at least once a week. Don't be intimidated if you've never made Vietnamese noodle soup. As a busy mom, My is a master of finding ways to take shortcuts in the kitchen—without taking shortcuts on flavor. Make this once and you'll have the hang of it for future fast pho.

VEGETARIAN PHO

Serves 4

1 (14-ounce) block firm tofu, drained and pressed (see Tip)

1½ tablespoons coconut oil

12 cups vegetable broth

1 ounce star anise (about 4 pods)

2 ounces grated peeled fresh ginger (about 2 tablespoons)

4 garlic cloves, smashed and peeled

½ medium white onion, diced

1 teaspoon sea salt, plus more as needed

1½ teaspoons light soy sauce

1 tablespoon toasted sesame oil

8 ounces rice noodles

2 cups sliced shiitake mushrooms

4 medium heads baby bok choy, quartered lengthwise

+

DAIRY-FREE

GLUTEN-FREE

LOW-INFLAMMATION

VEGAN

VEGETARIAN

BETTER DIGESTION

TO SERVE

Fresh Thai basil leaves

Fresh lime juice

Hoisin sauce

Sriracha

Tip: To drain your tofu, pat it dry, wrap it in paper towels, then set it on a plate with another heavy plate or other object on top. Let it sit for at least 15 minutes before cooking.

1. Slice the tofu into 8 thin rectangular pieces.

2. Melt the coconut oil in a large skillet over medium-high heat. When it shimmers, add the tofu and fry for 3 to 5 minutes per side, until crispy and golden brown on both sides.

3. In a large stockpot, combine the broth, star anise, ginger, garlic, onion, salt, soy sauce, and sesame oil. Bring to a boil over high heat, then reduce the heat to low, and simmer, with the lid ajar, for 30 minutes, or until the flavors have melded.

4. Meanwhile, in a separate large pot, bring 10 cups water to a boil over high heat. Dunk the rice noodles into the boiling water for 30 seconds, just until softened, then drain. Divide the noodles among four bowls.

5. Using a slotted spoon, transfer all the solid ingredients from the broth to a medium bowl and cover, leaving only the clear broth in the pot. Add the shiitakes and bok choy to the broth. Season with a generous pinch of salt and cook until the bok choy and shiitakes start to wilt slightly.

6. Divide the cooked vegetables, fried tofu, and hot broth evenly among the bowls. Top each with Thai basil leaves, lime juice, hoisin, and sriracha and serve hot.

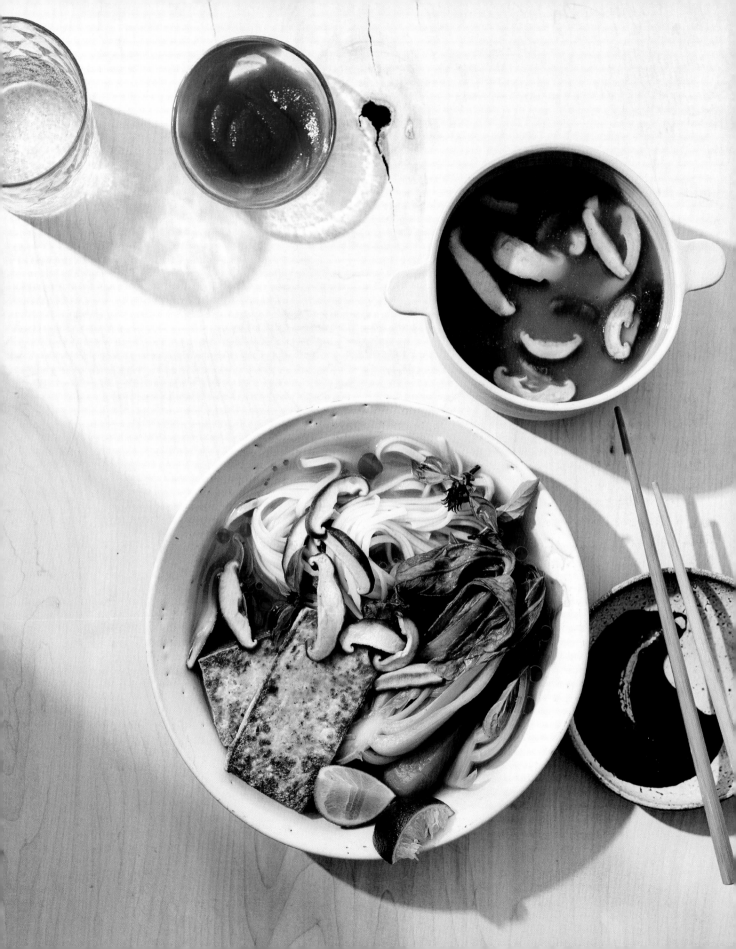

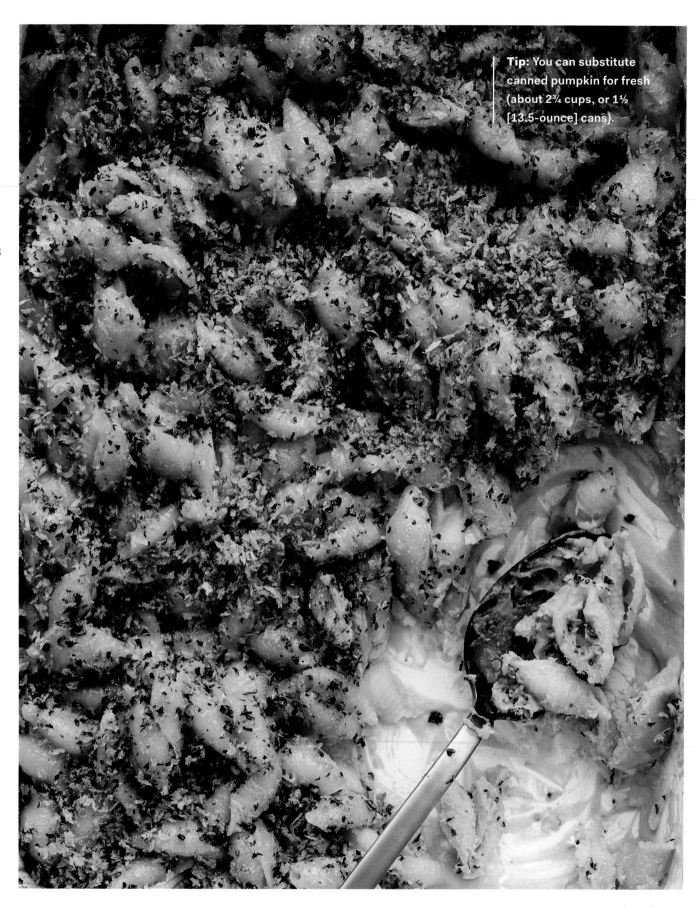

Tip: You can substitute canned pumpkin for fresh (about 2¾ cups, or 1½ [13.5-ounce] cans).

CANDICE KUMAI

Years of culinary school and cooking on the line at restaurants inspired wellness It-girl Candice Kumai to create playful recipes with fresh produce, devotion—and an edge—for making at home. "I'm proof that you can have it all—mac and cheese and gut-healthy miso all in one!" says the cookbook author, podcast host, and Well+Good Council member. She adds miso paste to this comforting dish for a probiotic punch and extra nutritional yeast on top for a crunchy, creamy bake that will blow your mind. "People can never believe coconut and butternut squash could be this freaking good," says Candice.

VEGAN PUMPKIN MAC + CHEESE

Serves 8

Coconut oil spray

1 medium pumpkin, peeled, seeded, and chopped into 1-inch cubes (or see Tip)

4 to 6 garlic cloves, peeled

2 sprigs thyme

2¾ cups coconut milk (about 1½ [13.5-ounce] cans)

3 tablespoons white miso paste

Sea salt

4 cups uncooked pasta shells or penne

Freshly ground black pepper

¼ cup nutritional yeast

FOR THE CRUMB TOPPING

½ cup panko bread crumbs

1 tablespoon garlic powder

¼ teaspoon sea salt

½ cup finely chopped kale or fresh parsley leaves

2 tablespoons nutritional yeast (optional)

1. Preheat the oven to 375°F. Lightly coat a 9 by 13-inch baking dish with cooking spray.

2. In a large saucepan, combine the pumpkin, garlic, thyme, coconut milk, and miso. Season with salt. Cook over medium heat, stirring occasionally, until the pumpkin is fork-tender, about 30 minutes. Be sure to keep the pumpkin submerged in liquid, adding 1 tablespoon of water if necessary. Discard the thyme sprigs. Carefully transfer the mixture to a high-speed blender or food processor and blend until completely smooth.

3. Meanwhile, bring a large pot of water to a boil over high heat. Salt the water, add the pasta, and cook according to the package directions until just al dente. Drain and rinse with cool water.

4. Spread the pasta in the prepared pan and pour the pumpkin purée over the top. Season with salt and pepper, then gently fold in the nutritional yeast. Mix well to combine, ensuring that all the noodles are coated. Cover the dish with aluminum foil and bake for about 25 minutes, or until bubbling and cooked through.

5. Meanwhile, make the crumb topping. In a small bowl, stir together the bread crumbs, garlic powder, sea salt, kale, and nutritional yeast (if using).

6. Remove the pasta from the oven and turn the broiler to high. Uncover the baking dish and sprinkle the bread crumb topping all over. Broil for about 2 minutes, or until the topping is golden brown.

7. Serve warm, family-style. Store the leftovers in an airtight container in the refrigerator for up to 5 days.

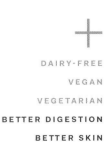

DAIRY-FREE

VEGAN

VEGETARIAN

BETTER DIGESTION

BETTER SKIN

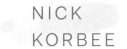

Chef Nick Korbee biked three hundred miles in three days the week he created this recipe for Egg Shop, his trendy NYC café that's obsessed with—you guessed it—egg dishes. In addition to helping him dream up a salad packed with healthy fats and protein, the distance he logged helped raise $1.5 million for No Kid Hungry to give children better meals at school as part of the Chefs Cycle campaign. The fit foodie says "healthy eating is about the relationship between the body, soul, and community," and, no surprise, Nick's sense of commitment extends to food. He makes the whitefish salad in-house, but you have our full permission to head to the store.

160

WHITEFISH NIÇOISE SALAD

Serves 2

FOR THE POTATOES

1 tablespoon champagne vinegar or apple cider vinegar

2 tablespoons whole-grain mustard

1 tablespoon honey

3 tablespoons prepared horseradish, or 1 tablespoon grated fresh horseradish

¼ cup olive oil

1 pound red potatoes, blanched

¼ cup thinly sliced fresh chives

1 teaspoon sea salt

Freshly ground black pepper

FOR THE SALAD

2 heads Bibb or Little Gem lettuce, coarsely chopped

Pinch of caraway seeds, toasted

½ cup niçoise olives, pitted

¼ cup pickled red onion

2 tablespoons capers

8 ounces French string beans, blanched

2 large hard-boiled eggs, halved

4 tablespoons store-bought whitefish salad

Juice of ½ lemon (about 1 tablespoon)

¼ cup fresh dill, or to taste

1. Make the potatoes. In a medium bowl, whisk together the vinegar, mustard, honey, horseradish, and olive oil. Add the potatoes to the bowl and toss with the chives and sea salt. Season with pepper.

2. Assemble the salad. Divide the salad between two plates. Place half of the lettuce, horseradish potatoes, caraway seeds, olives, pickled onion, capers, and string beans on each plate. Top each with a hard-boiled egg and 2 tablespoons of the whitefish salad. Finish with the lemon juice and dill.

DAIRY-FREE

GLUTEN-FREE

LOW-INFLAMMATION

BETTER ENERGY

BETTER FOCUS

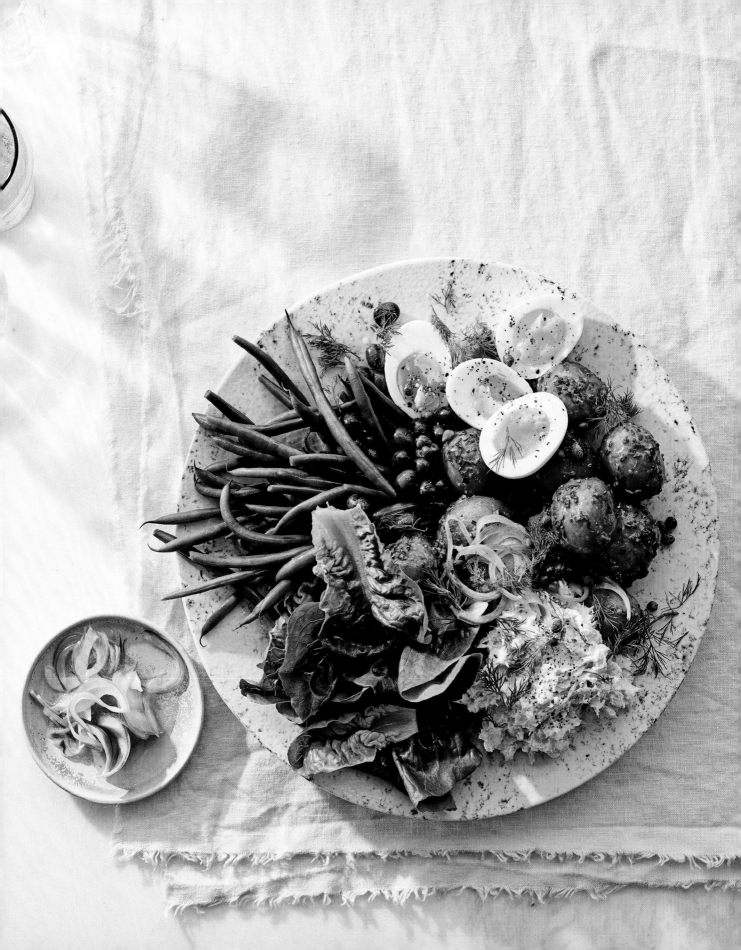

EAT FOR BETTER ENERGY

Forget about coffee, tea, and caffeine for a hot minute. While sippable stimulants might be the first thing that comes to mind when you need a shot of energy, especially first thing in the morning, eating healthy foods that can give you energy—and there are a lot of them—is a solid long-term plan. (But, yes, you can keep your latte, too.)

As a dietitian in functional nutrition, I've spent the past decade coaching women to feel their best by explaining the science behind food. There's been a common theme in their desires to feel healthier: "I want more energy!" No one feels like they have enough fuel in their tank. And most of them are probably right. Feeling sluggish or having dips in energy has (sadly!) become commonplace. Everyone's become intimately aware of how poor sleep, stress, anxiety, and our always-on lifestyles can make us feel depleted. But that feeling also stems from what you put on your plate.

Many energy-boosting beverages and grab-and-go snacks are overly processed and high in oils, sodium, and added sugars. (Take a close look at the ingredients of many protein bars and energy drinks.) Heck, yes, they'll put a pep in your step and keep you coming back for more—studies have pointed to sugar's cocaine-like addictive properties in the body—but these faux foods aren't really your friends. They're just loaning you something you could own.

The key to feeling revved up and recharged by what you eat—versus feeling exhausted, bloated, or unsatisfied—lies in cooking with nutrient-dense real foods, like produce and protein, and lowering your inflammation. You'll know these foods by their combination of protein, fiber, high-quality carbohydrates, good fats, minerals, vitamins, phytonutrients, and antioxidants. Your body uses these super-loaded foods as fuel, and eating them is a beautiful, synergistic way to keep your digestion humming, your focus sharp, and, yes, your energy buzzing.

The key to eating for energy is balance: eat healthy fats, protein (plant or animal), and fiber from veggies at each meal. Doing so can help balance your blood sugar and may help increase, or at least stabilize, your energy—win! Here's how to go about it, and a grocery list of nutrient-dense foods that will help power your undoubtedly super-busy life:

EAT YOUR FRUITS AND VEGETABLES. My favorite picks for fruits are berries, since they're loaded with the most nutrients and antioxidants, highest in fiber, and typically the lowest in sugar. You can't go wrong with any vegetable, but I recommend choosing the nonstarchy ones and dark leafy greens as often as possible. These foods are rich in phytonutrients, antioxidants, minerals, and vitamins, which are vital to energy.

HAVE A HIGH-QUALITY FAT WITH EVERY MEAL. Good fats, such as monounsaturated fatty acids and alpha-lipoic acid, help your body absorb and use fat-soluble nutrients (commonly found in plants) for energy. They also help lower inflammation. Good choices are olive oil, coconut oil, avocados, nuts, and seeds.

ADD ANTIOXIDANT-RICH FOODS TO YOUR DIET. Antioxidants help counterbalance oxidative stress and free radicals caused by a poor diet, stress, and more. These wreak havoc on your mitochondria, which are the battery packs of your cells that make all your energy. Blueberries, dark chocolate, and matcha are just a few foods that are especially high in antioxidants, although you'll find them in all fruits and vegetables.

GET YOUR CARBS FROM PLANTS. Whole-food carbohydrates in the form of sweet potatoes or other tubers, quinoa, millet, sourdough bread, legumes, and anything that comes from the earth are the best sources.

BUMP UP THE VITAMIN B. Dark leafy greens are high in vitamin B, as is nutritional yeast (one of my favorites), which is also a great source of protein and can be used in salads, stir-fries, or soups. Another superfood that can give you a boost of B vitamins is bee pollen, which you can get in many grocery stores or online.

—McKEL HILL, MS, RDN, LDN

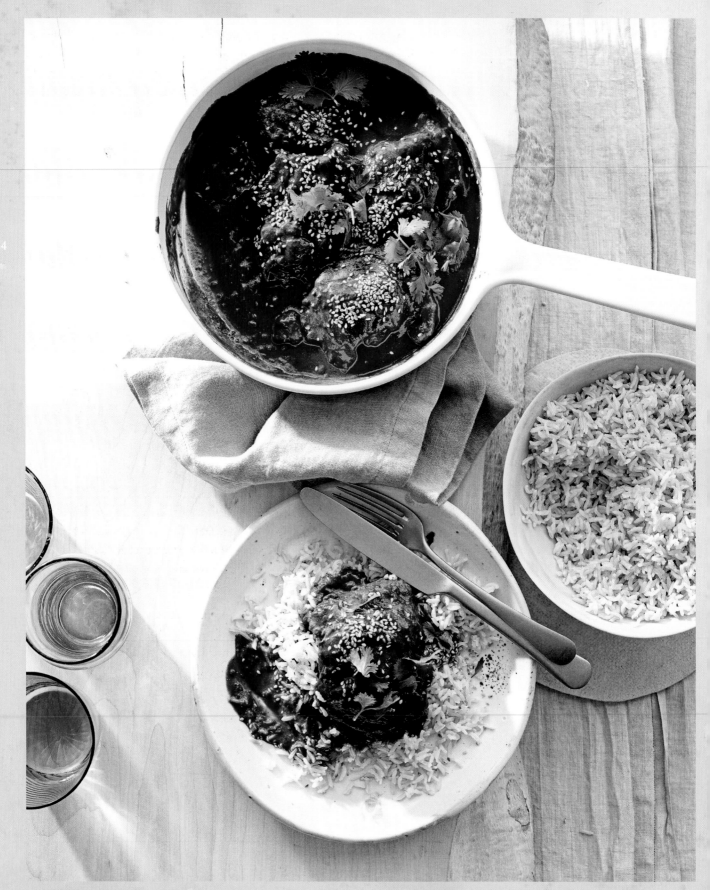

NICK
GREEN

Nick Green, cofounder of the organic online retailer Thrive Market, helped change the game when it comes to finding alt-ingredients online (think monk fruit sugar and almond flour), but the CEO is also a fan of tradition. "Food can evoke such great memories," says the social-impact entrepreneur. "My mother's family is Mexican American; this is a simplified, wholesome version of the dish she often prepared for us when we were kids." If you prefer your mole a little sweeter, try adding ground raisins.

CHICKEN WITH CHOCOLATE MOLE

Serves 4

FOR THE CHICKEN

1 to 1½ pounds boneless, skinless chicken thighs

Kosher salt and freshly ground black pepper

2 tablespoons coconut oil

FOR THE MOLE

1 small yellow onion, grated

½ teaspoon kosher salt

1 tablespoon chili powder

1 teaspoon garlic powder

½ teaspoon ground cumin

½ teaspoon ground cinnamon

⅛ teaspoon cayenne pepper

2 tablespoons tomato paste

1 cup chicken bone broth

¼ cup coarsely chopped dark chocolate (at least 72% cacao)

1 tablespoon almond butter

¼ cup raisins, ground (optional)

Chopped cilantro and toasted sesame seeds

Cooked brown rice

1. Make the chicken. Pat the chicken thighs very dry, then season both sides with ¼ teaspoon each of the salt and pepper.

2. Melt the coconut oil in a large cast-iron skillet over high heat. When it shimmers, using tongs, add the chicken in a single layer. Sear, without moving, for about 2 minutes, until the skin starts to brown, then flip and sear for about 2 minutes more, until beginning to brown on the second side. Transfer the chicken to a paper towel–lined plate to drain.

3. Make the mole. Add the onion to the same skillet and cook over medium heat, stirring, until soft and translucent, 4 to 5 minutes. Add the salt, chili powder, garlic powder, cumin, cinnamon, and cayenne and cook, stirring, until fragrant, about 30 seconds. Add the tomato paste, broth, chocolate, almond butter, and raisins (if using). Stir until the chocolate has melted, about 1 minute, then reduce the heat to medium-low and bring the mixture to a simmer.

4. Return the chicken to the skillet, nestling it into the mole. Cover and simmer until the chicken is completely cooked through, about 15 minutes. Transfer the chicken to a plate and cover loosely with aluminum foil to keep warm. Cook the sauce until it has reduced by about one-third, about 10 minutes more.

5. Top the chicken with the sauce. Garnish with the cilantro and sesame seeds. Serve family-style with brown rice.

DAIRY-FREE

GLUTEN-FREE

KETOGENIC

LOW-INFLAMMATION

PALEO

BETTER DIGESTION

Genius Foods author Max Lugavere spent the better half of a decade learning all there is to know about the human brain, but long before that, while in college in Miami, he focused on consuming as much Cuban food as he could. "Especially *picadillo*," says the health and science journalist, who argues in his work that grass-fed, organic red meat can be a brain-boosting food, if eaten in moderation. This Paleo take on the traditional Cuban dish is one Max makes on the reg. For some anti-inflammatory action, drizzle a little extra-virgin olive oil on top.

GRASS-FED PICADILLO

Serves 4

1 tablespoon extra-virgin olive oil

1 large yellow onion, finely chopped

4 garlic cloves, smashed
and peeled

1 pound ground beef

1 teaspoon sea salt

1½ teaspoons freshly ground
black pepper

¼ teaspoon crushed red pepper
flakes (optional)

1 cup tomato sauce

½ cup pitted green olives, sliced

1 teaspoon ground cumin

1. Heat the olive oil in a large skillet over medium heat. When it shimmers, add the onion and cook for 4 to 5 minutes, until softened. Add the garlic and cook until fragrant, about 1 minute.

2. Add the ground beef, salt, black pepper, and red pepper flakes (if using). Cook, breaking up the meat with a wooden spoon as it cooks, for about 10 minutes, or until browned and cooked through. Add the tomato sauce, olives, and cumin. Reduce the heat to low and simmer for 10 minutes, or until the flavors have melded.

3. Remove from the heat and serve warm.

DAIRY-FREE

GLUTEN-FREE

KETOGENIC

PALEO

BETTER ENERGY

BETTER FOCUS

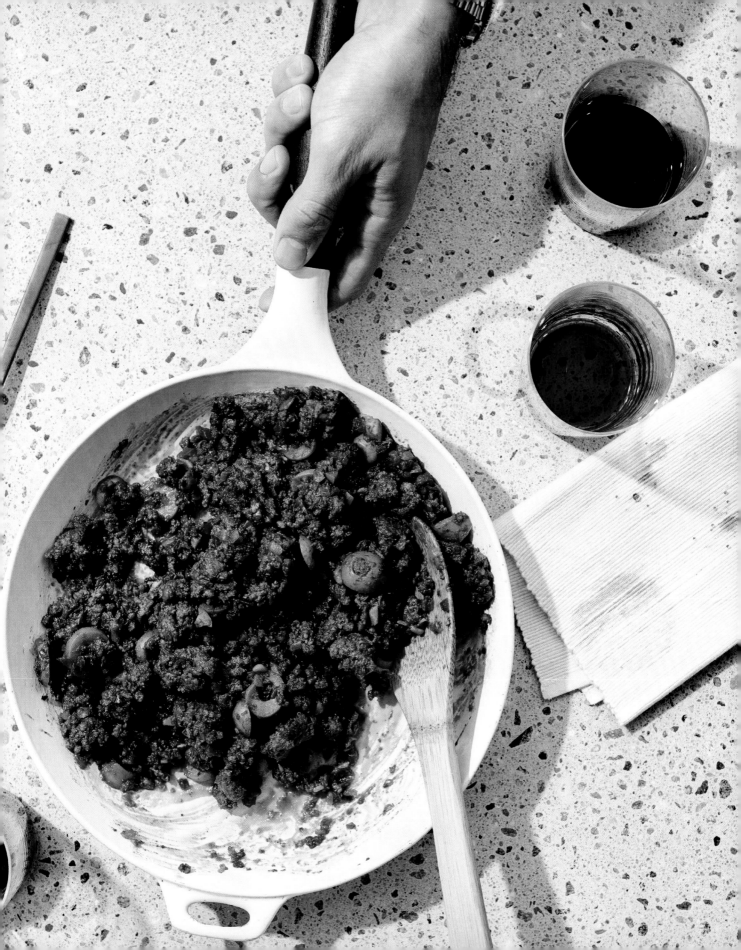

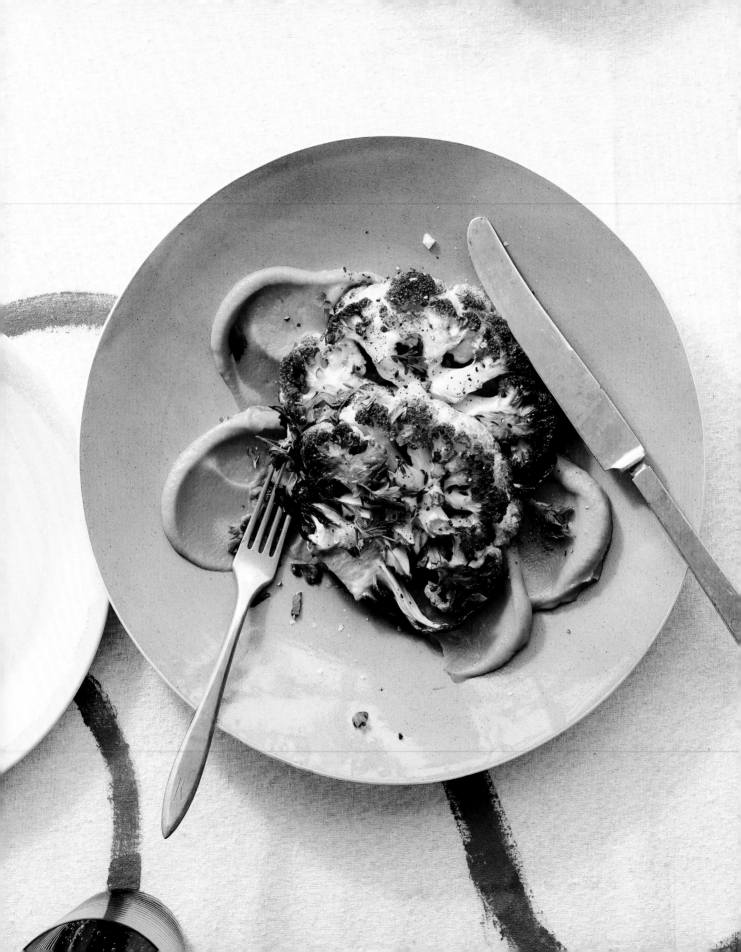

KIMBERLY
SNYDER

Well+Good Council member Kimberly Snyder, CN, created this easy entrée—combining a streak of bright orange with pops of green—as an aesthetically (and crowd!) pleasing way to feature everyone's obsession, cauliflower, as the main attraction. "Plus, cumin, turmeric, and cinnamon are digestion-enhancing spices," says the *Radical Beauty* best-selling author and wellness expert. "Which makes it nourishing for your body, energy, and soul." Kimberly also notes cauliflower's skin-bettering properties, in case you needed another reason to add this dish to your mood board.

FEEL-GOOD CAULIFLOWER STEAKS
WITH BETA-CAROTENE PUREE

Serves 4

FOR THE CAULIFLOWER

1 head of cauliflower

¼ cup coconut oil, melted

1 tablespoon lemon juice

1 tablespoon cumin

Sea salt, to taste

Freshly ground black pepper, to taste

FOR THE PUREE

3 medium carrots, sliced into thick chunks

1 medium sweet potato, peeled and coarsely chopped

2 to 3 tablespoons coconut milk

¼ teaspoon turmeric

½ teaspoon cinnamon

⅛ teaspoon sea salt, or to taste

½ cup parsley chopped, for topping

1. Preheat oven to 400° F. Line a baking sheet with parchment paper.

2. Slice the cauliflower through the core into 4 "steaks." Place the cauliflower steaks on the prepared baking sheet.

3. Whisk the coconut oil, lemon juice, cumin, sea salt, and black pepper together in a bowl. Brush ½ of the coconut oil mixture over the tops of the cauliflower steaks.

4. Roast cauliflower steaks in the oven for 15 minutes. Gently turn over each steak and brush with remaining coconut oil mixture. Continue roasting 15 to 20 minutes more, until tender and golden.

5. Meanwhile, place the carrots and sweet potatoes in a medium-sized pot and cover with cold water. Bring to a boil and cook for 20 minutes, until the carrots are very tender.

6. Drain the carrots and sweet potatoes and put them in the food processor with 2 tablespoons of coconut milk, along with the turmeric, cinnamon, and sea salt. Puree on high until smooth. Stop occasionally to push the contents to the bottom. If necessary, add a bit more coconut milk to thin out the puree, but the less liquid, the better.

7. To assemble, spread ¼ of the puree (or less if you prefer it to be just a streak of color) on the bottom of each of four plates. Top with the cauliflower steaks and sprinkle with fresh parsley. This is great to serve along with or after a big green salad.

+

DAIRY-FREE

GLUTEN-FREE

LOW-INFLAMMATION

VEGAN

VEGETARIAN

BETTER DIGESTION

BETTER MOOD

BETTER SKIN

Superstar athlete Venus Williams doesn't have a ton of time to spend in the kitchen, considering that she's always on the road for tennis tournaments (or running her activewear line, overseeing her interior design business, or generally being a total boss). "But when I do cook, I love a vegan burrito inspired by one of my favorite restaurants—Christopher's Kitchen in Palm Beach," says the Wimbledon champ. "It's delicious and keeps me energized even through the toughest workouts." The jalapeño cashew cream kicks it up to a professional level, making this dish deserving of a trophy of its own. Follow the recipe exactly for meal-prepping burritos to freeze.

JALAPEÑO VEGAN BURRITO

Serves 4

2 teaspoons olive oil

1 small red onion, diced

1 large red bell pepper, cut into ¼-inch dice

1 garlic clove, minced

1 cup sliced button or cremini mushrooms

1 cup cooked jasmine or brown rice

1 cup canned black beans, drained and rinsed

Sea salt

4 whole-wheat tortillas

2 cups shredded romaine lettuce

1 cup guacamole

1 cup tomato salsa

¼ cup Jalapeño Cashew Cream (recipe follows)

DAIRY-FREE

VEGAN

VEGETARIAN

BETTER ENERGY

BETTER FOCUS

1. Heat the olive oil in a large skillet over medium heat. When it shimmers, add the onion, bell pepper, and garlic. Cook, stirring occasionally, until the vegetables are soft and just beginning to color, about 3 minutes. Transfer to a medium bowl.

2. Add the mushrooms to the skillet, increase the heat to medium-high, and cook until soft, about 2 minutes. Transfer the mushrooms to the bowl with the other vegetables. Stir in the rice and black beans and season with salt.

3. To assemble the burritos, lay out the tortillas on a clean surface. Divide the vegetable-rice mixture evenly among the tortillas, spooning it neatly down the centers. Top with the lettuce, using about ½ cup on each. Spoon the guacamole and salsa over the top, using about ¼ cup on each. Drizzle with the cashew cream.

4. Tuck in the two sides of the tortillas and, starting from the edge closest to you, roll them up gently but with some pressure to create a neat log. Slice them in half across the middle and serve.

JALAPEÑO CASHEW CREAM

Makes about 2 cups

2 cups raw cashews, soaked in water overnight and drained

½ to 1 medium jalapeño, sliced

Juice of ½ lemon (about 1 tablespoon)

Kosher salt

1. In a high-speed blender or food processor, combine the soaked cashews, jalapeño, lemon juice, and salt to taste. Blend until smooth; add 1 tablespoon water, if needed, to reach the desired consistency.

2. Store the cashew cream in an airtight container in the refrigerator for up to 3 days.

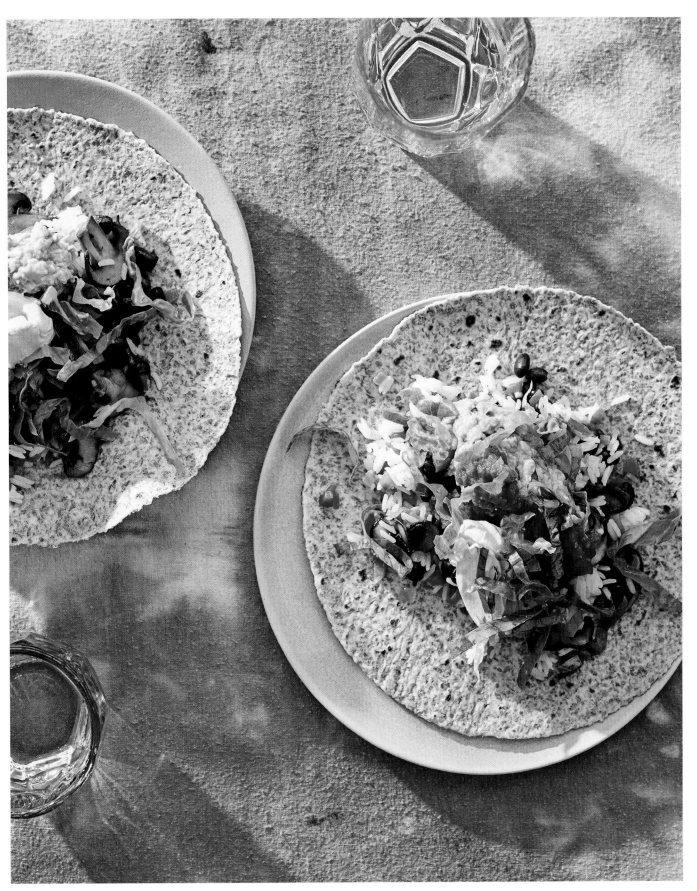

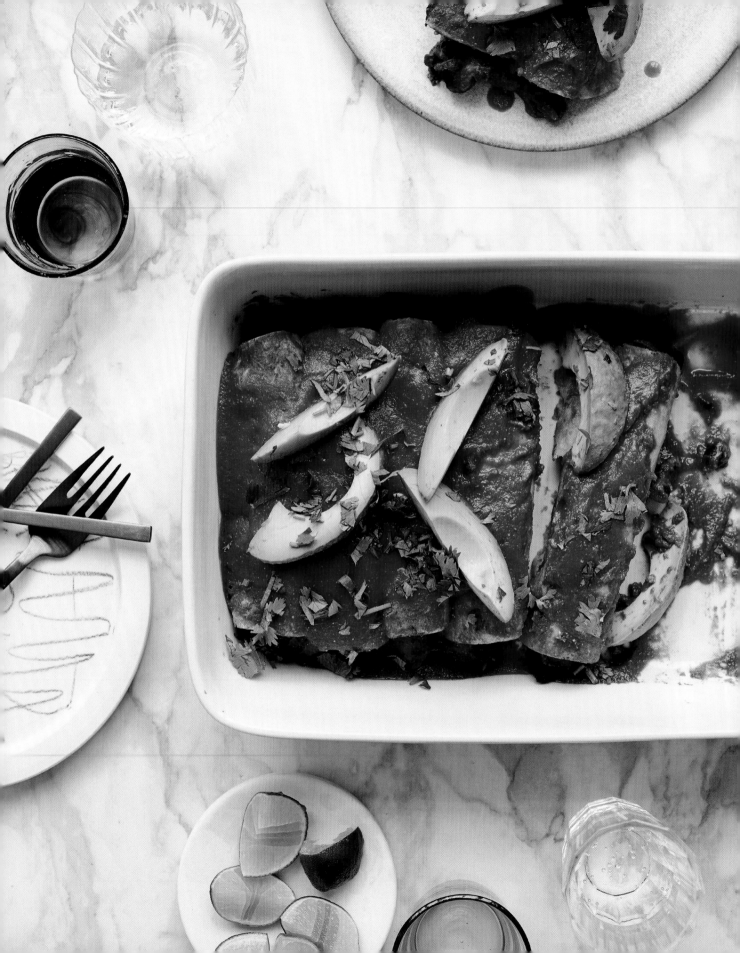

Wendy Lopez is a meal-prep queen. As the cofounder of Food Heaven Made Easy—the multimedia healthy-food brand she runs with fellow registered dietitian (and BFF) Jess Jones—she shares brilliant intel for getting plant-based meals on the table each night with minimal time in the kitchen. Wendy makes this veggie-packed dish to ease her cooking load throughout the week. "It's the ideal intersection of comfort food and nutritious ingredients," she says, noting its protein, fiber, and iron content. These enchiladas are also easy to customize: Try them with kale, chard, or even scrambled eggs for a breakfast-for-dinner twist.

CREAMY CASHEW–BLACK BEAN ENCHILADAS

Serves 4

FOR THE FILLING

½ cup raw cashews, soaked in water for at least 1 hour or up to overnight and drained

2 cups cooked or canned black beans, drained and rinsed

1 teaspoon olive oil

¼ red onion, minced

1 jalapeño, seeded and chopped

3 cups coarsely chopped button mushrooms

1 teaspoon paprika

½ teaspoon ground cumin

Sea salt

FOR THE SAUCE

1 cup vegetable broth

1 cup tomato sauce

1 teaspoon ground cumin

1 teaspoon garlic powder

1 canned chipotle pepper in adobo sauce

TO ASSEMBLE

8 corn tortillas

Chopped cilantro, sliced avocado, and black pepper

1. Preheat the oven to 350°F.

2. Make the filling. In a food processor, combine the cashews, 1 cup of the black beans, and ⅓ cup water. Process until a paste forms.

3. Heat the olive oil in a medium pot over medium heat. When it shimmers, add the onion and jalapeño and cook, stirring, until slightly softened, 1 to 2 minutes. Add the mushrooms, cover, and cook until the mushrooms are beginning to brown and release some liquid, 2 to 3 minutes. Add the cashew-bean paste, the paprika, cumin, and remaining 1 cup black beans and stir to combine. Reduce the heat to low and cook for 2 to 3 minutes, until the mixture begins to thin. Season with salt and remove the pot from the heat.

4. Make the sauce. In a blender or food processor, combine the broth, tomato sauce, cumin, garlic powder, and chipotle. Blend until smooth.

5. Assemble the enchiladas. Working in batches, place the tortillas in a large skillet over high heat and cook for 1 minute per side, until browned and pliable. Remove from the heat and lightly dip them into the sauce. Fill the center of each tortilla with the filling and roll gently to keep the filling inside, placing them seam-side down in rows in an 11 by 7-inch baking dish. Pour half the sauce over the top.

6. Bake for 25 minutes, or until the tops of the enchiladas begin to brown. Pour the remaining sauce over the top. Add cilantro and avocado, and season with black pepper. Serve warm, family style.

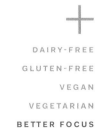

DAIRY-FREE

GLUTEN-FREE

VEGAN

VEGETARIAN

BETTER FOCUS

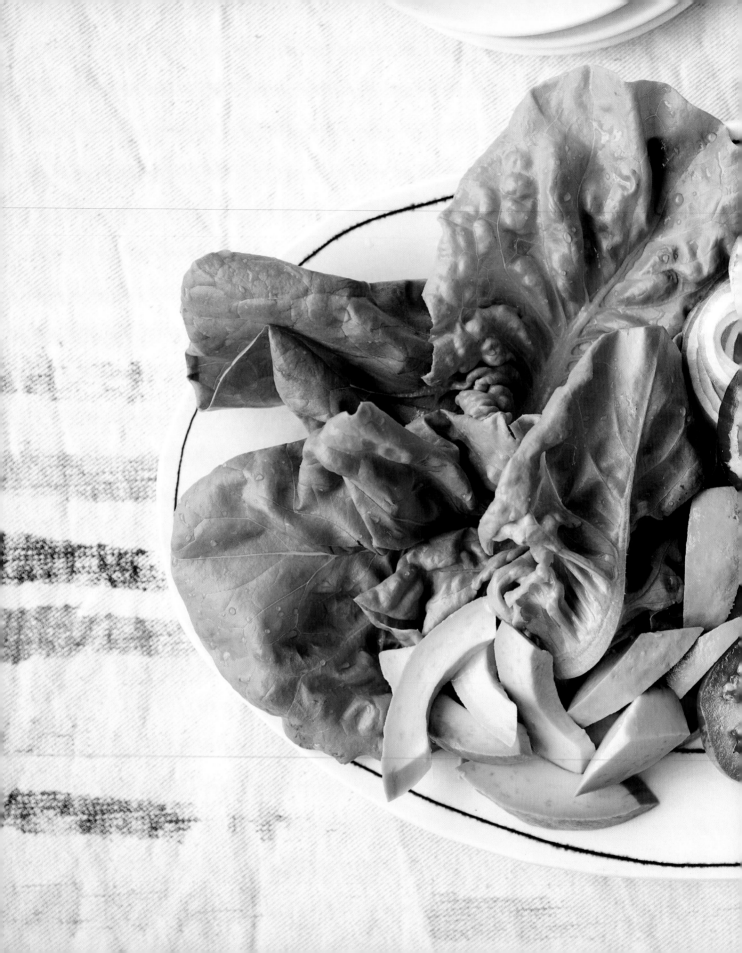

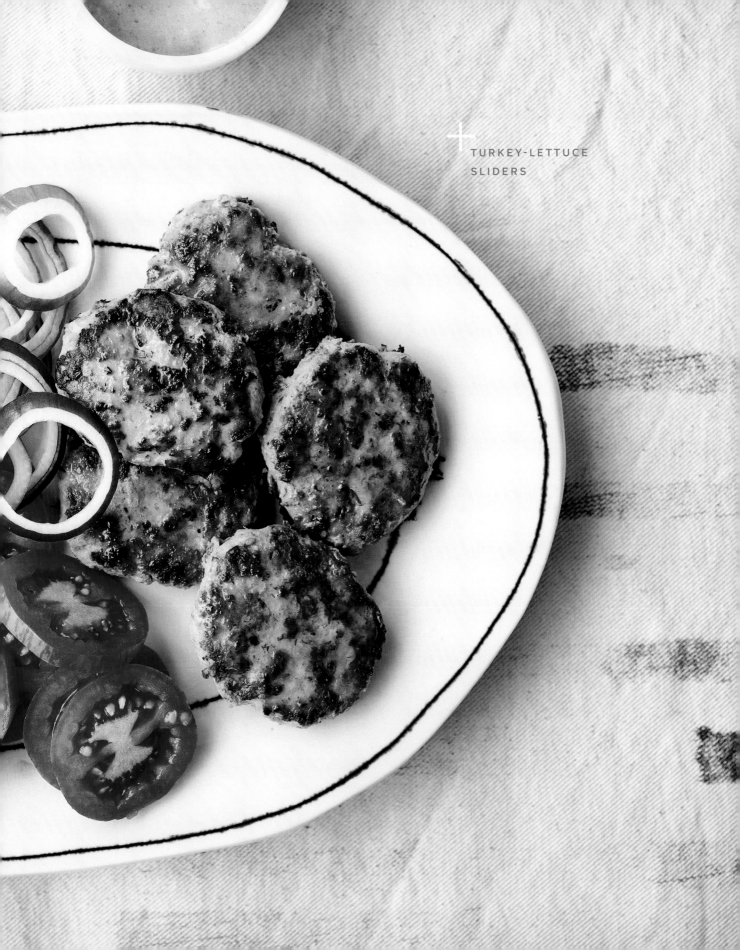

Body by Simone founder Simone De La Rue, who seems to have trained half of Hollywood at this point (everyone from Jennifer Garner to Reese Witherspoon), maintains her infectious energy by keeping her diet simple. Her motto is to think like a cavewoman, mostly sticking to the Paleo diet. "I look at food as something to fulfill and sustain you, not something that serves as a reward or source of guilt," the former Broadway dancer says. She whips up these lettuce wraps for a quick, protein-heavy lunch to fuel her jam-packed days and intense workouts.

TURKEY-LETTUCE SLIDERS

Make 10 to 12 sliders

1 pound lean or extra-lean ground turkey

1 large egg, beaten

1½ teaspoons garlic powder

¾ teaspoon pink Himalayan salt

1 tablespoon minced red onion

1 tablespoon chopped fresh parsley

¼ teaspoon freshly ground black pepper

1 teaspoon olive oil

6 large Bibb lettuce leaves, torn in half

Sliced onion, tomato, and avocado, or your favorite toppings, for serving

1. In a medium bowl, combine the turkey, egg, garlic powder, salt, onion, parsley, and pepper. Using a wooden spoon, mix to incorporate evenly. With clean hands, form the mixture into ten to twelve ½-inch-thick patties.

2. Heat the olive oil in a large skillet over medium-high heat. When it shimmers, working in batches to avoid overcrowding the pan, add the patties and cook for 2 to 4 minutes per side, until no longer pink in the center.

3. Place one patty on each lettuce leaf half. Serve open-faced with onion, tomato, and avocado, or your favorite toppings.

DAIRY-FREE

GLUTEN-FREE

KETOGENIC

LOW-INFLAMMATION

PALEO

BETTER SKIN

BETTER SLEEP

When she lived in New York City's East Village, holistic digestive health expert Robyn Youkilis was frequently tempted by the delicious-looking Vietnamese food on basically every corner. Instead of giving in to takeout on the regular, she found a way to enjoy a classic bánh mì in a way that pleases her taste buds *and* her gut. How? By loading it up with lots of vegetables and not one, but *two* fermented foods. "Go with your gut," says the health coach, author, and speaker. "Learning to listen to our bodies will lead us to exactly the foods, workouts, and life choices that are best for us in each moment."

GO-WITH-YOUR-GUT BÁNH MÌ

Serves 2 or 3

¼ teaspoon crushed red pepper flakes

2 tablespoons toasted sesame oil

2 tablespoons almond butter or peanut butter

2 tablespoons tamari or coconut aminos

Juice of 1 lime

3 tablespoons pure maple syrup

8 to 10 ounces tempeh, cut into 1-inch triangles

Coconut oil spray

TO ASSEMBLE

5 or 6 collard green leaves, thick stems removed

2 to 3 tablespoons spicy mayonnaise

1 small seedless cucumber, cut into small matchsticks

2 store-bought fermented carrot sticks, thinly sliced

2 scallions, sliced

3 tablespoons chopped fresh cilantro and/or parsley

2 to 3 teaspoons black sesame seeds

1. In a medium bowl, combine the red pepper flakes, sesame oil, almond butter, tamari, lime juice, and maple syrup until well incorporated. Add the tempeh, cover, and marinate for 1 hour at room temperature or up to overnight in the refrigerator. (Alternatively, pour the marinade into a zip-top bag, add the tempeh, seal, and marinate as directed.)

2. Preheat the oven to 375°F. Line a baking sheet with parchment paper and coat the parchment with coconut oil spray.

3. Arrange the tempeh on the prepared baking sheet in an even layer, reserving the marinade. Bake for 20 to 30 minutes, until golden brown and caramelized.

4. Meanwhile, transfer the remaining marinade to a small saucepan. Cook over low heat, stirring occasionally to prevent scorching, until reduced by one-quarter, about 10 minutes.

5. Remove the baking sheet from the oven and brush the tempeh with the reduced marinade.

6. To assemble, lay the collard leaves on a flat surface. Spread the spicy mayo over each leaf. Layer the tempeh, sliced cucumber, fermented carrots, scallions, cilantro and/or parsley, and sesame seeds on top of each, keeping the toppings on just one half. Roll up the collard leaves, folding up the bottom first to keep all the toppings in, then folding in one side, then the other, and tightly rolling to the top. Enjoy immediately.

+

DAIRY-FREE

GLUTEN-FREE

VEGETARIAN

BETTER DIGESTION

BETTER ENERGY

BETTER SLEEP

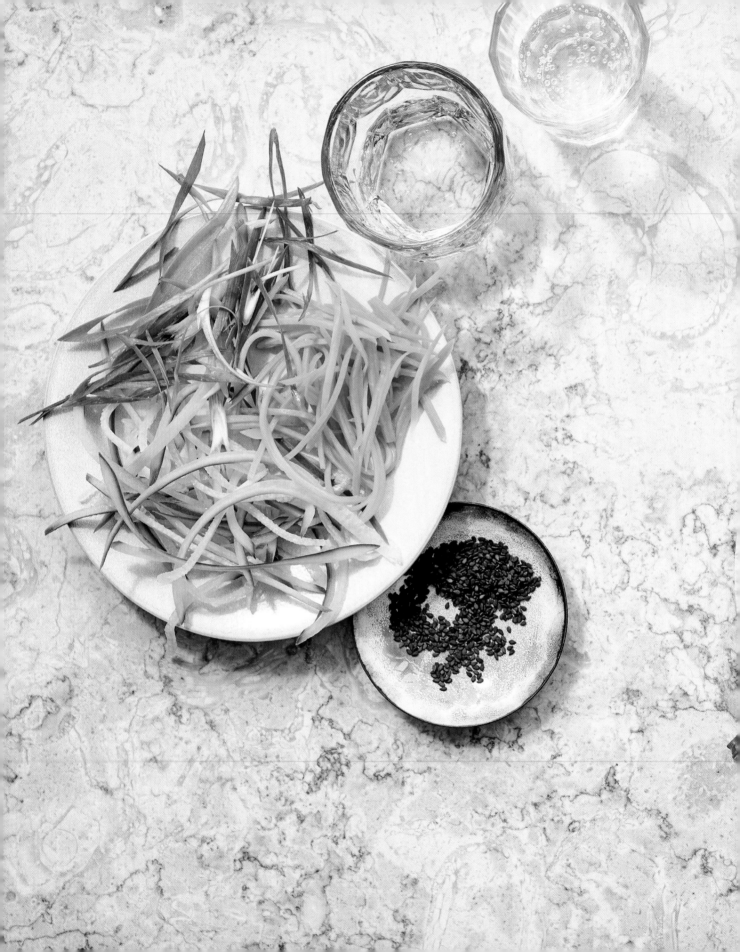

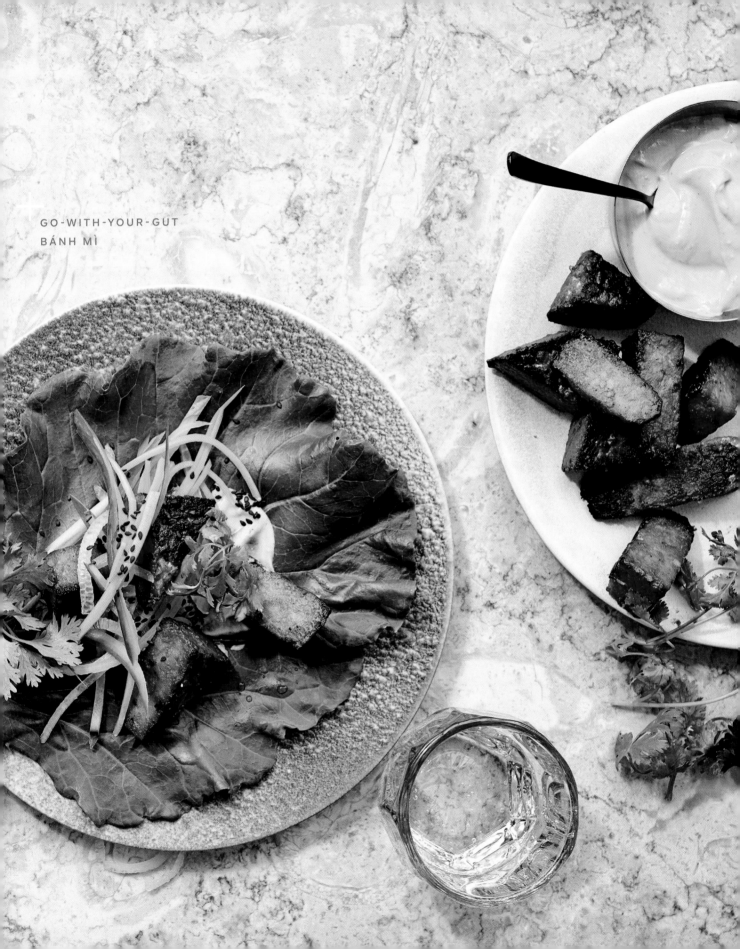

GO-WITH-YOUR-GUT
BÁNH MÌ

"We all love the tasty comfort of a chicken tender," says Kelly LeVeque, a holistic nutritionist, wellness expert, and health coach who's worked with celebs like Jessica Alba and Molly Sims. This smart take on the classic adds a bump of healthy fat and fiber to the versatile, kid-approved dish standard, and makes meal-prepping a breeze. "I believe in real food, real ingredients, and a clean diet," says the author of *Body Love*. At home, Kelly serves these impossibly juicy-on-the-inside, crunchy-on-the-outside chicken tenders with an avocado hummus, but they're the perfect partner for salads, pasta, grain bowls, and more.

CHIA + FLAX CHICKEN TENDERS

Serves 4 to 6

1 cup potato starch

1 teaspoon pink Himalayan salt

1 teaspoon freshly ground black pepper

2 large eggs

1 cup chia seeds

1 cup flaxseed

1 cup gluten-free panko bread crumbs or grain-free flour

2 teaspoons paprika

2 teaspoons garlic salt

Pinch of chopped fresh parsley

4 to 6 ounces uncooked chicken tenders, pounded to ½-inch thickness or less

¼ cup ghee

1. Preheat the oven to 350°F. Line a baking sheet with aluminum foil.

2. Create dredging stations: On a large plate, combine the potato starch, pink Himalayan salt, and pepper. In a shallow bowl, whisk the eggs. On a separate large plate, combine the chia, flaxseed, bread crumbs, paprika, garlic salt, and parsley.

3. One at a time, coat each chicken tender, first dipping it into the potato starch mixture, then into the egg mixture to coat completely, letting the excess drip off, then into the chia-flax mixture, pressing to adhere. Set the dredged piece on the prepared baking sheet and repeat to coat the remaining chicken.

4. Melt the ghee in a large skillet over medium heat. When it shimmers, working in batches to avoid overcrowding the skillet, add the chicken tenders and increase the heat to medium-high. Cook for 2 to 4 minutes, then use tongs to gently turn the tenders and cook for 2 to 4 minutes on the second side, until the coating is crisped and browned on both sides. Transfer the cooked tenders to a baking sheet as you finish each batch.

5. Transfer the tenders to the oven and bake for 10 to 12 minutes, until the chicken is completely cooked through. Serve warm with your favorite dip or side.

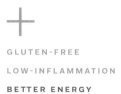

GLUTEN-FREE

LOW-INFLAMMATION

BETTER ENERGY

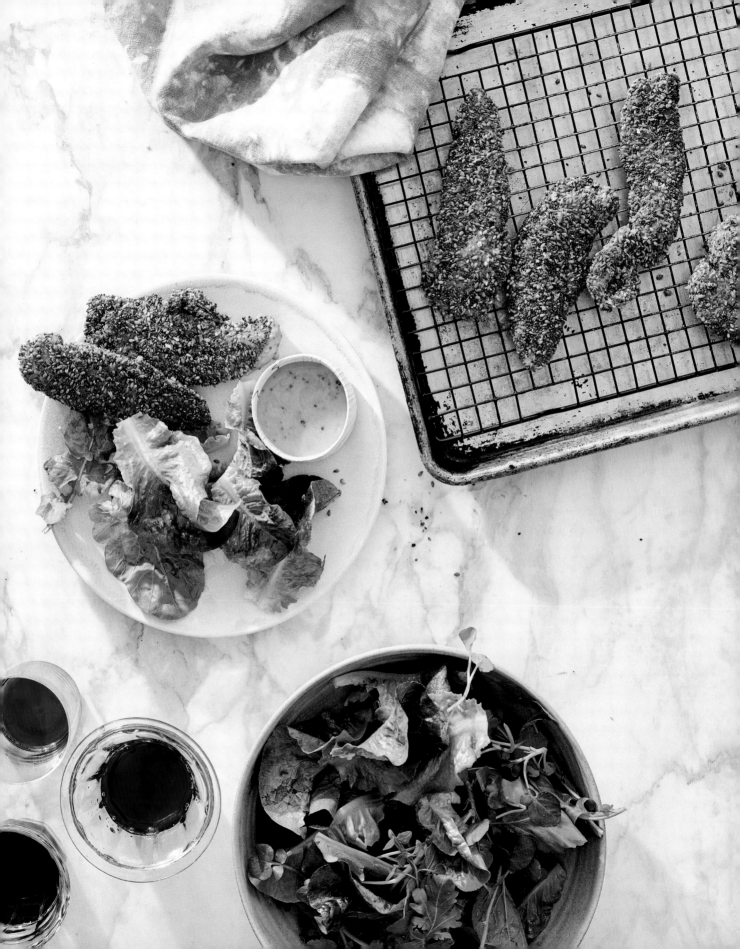

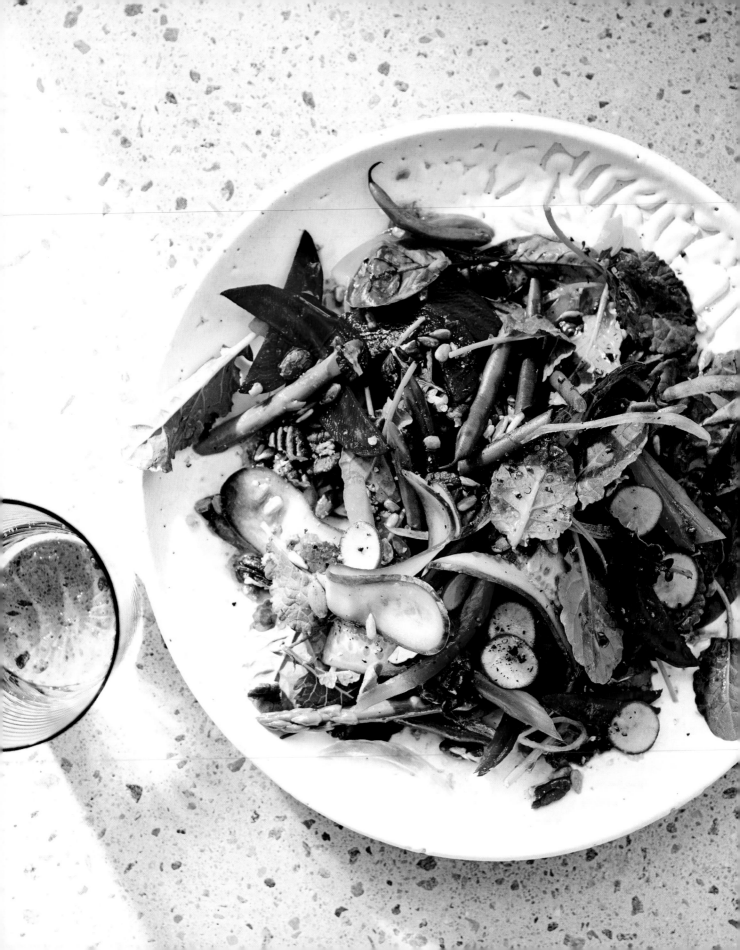

JILLIAN WRIGHT

Skin-health expert and Well+Good Council member Jillian Wright takes a minimalist approach to her daily beauty regimen—and you can see that focus on essentials in her approach to food, too. "I only put what is necessary in and on my body," says the trained esthetician and cofounder of Indie Beauty Expo. Jillian combines fresh ingredients (like asparagus and cucumber) for a happier digestive system and hydrated skin, which helps aid a full-body reset. "Eating this salad keeps me glowing," she says. Raw beet haters, beware: The delicious added crunch is about to change the way you think about the earthy red root.

10-INGREDIENT RESET SALAD

Serves 2 to 4

FOR THE DRESSING

1 garlic clove, minced

3 tablespoons balsamic vinegar

½ cup olive oil

Minced fresh peeled ginger

Ground turmeric

Pink Himalayan salt and freshly ground black pepper

FOR THE SALAD

2 tablespoons pink Himalayan salt

8 ounces asparagus (6 to 8 spears), woody ends removed

8 ounces haricots verts, trimmed

5 ounces greens, such as kale, spinach, or chard (1 medium bunch)

1 or 2 radishes, thinly sliced

½ medium cucumber, seeded and peeled into strips

1 or 2 red beets, peeled and sliced

1 or 2 tablespoons raw sunflower or pumpkin seeds

½ orange bell pepper, thinly sliced

¼ cup diced sweet onion

¼ cup chopped roasted pecans

1. Make the dressing. In a small bowl, whisk together the garlic, vinegar, and olive oil and season with ginger, turmeric, salt, and pepper to taste. Set aside until ready to serve.

2. Make the salad. In a medium pot, combine 8 cups water and the salt and bring to a boil over high heat. Fill a large bowl with ice and water and set it nearby. Add the asparagus and haricots verts to the boiling water and blanch until bright green, 2 to 3 minutes. Using tongs, transfer the vegetables to the ice water and let cool completely.

3. Drain the cooled asparagus and haricots verts and slice as desired.

4. In a medium bowl, combine the asparagus, haricots verts, greens, radishes, cucumber, beets, sunflower seeds, bell pepper, onion, and pecans. Add the dressing and toss until thoroughly combined.

5. Serve the salad family style, or store in an airtight glass container in the refrigerator for up to 3 days.

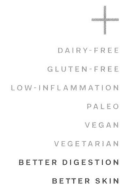

DAIRY-FREE

GLUTEN-FREE

LOW-INFLAMMATION

PALEO

VEGAN

VEGETARIAN

BETTER DIGESTION

BETTER SKIN

Food blogger Rens Kroes comes from a lineage in the Netherlands that includes an organic farmer, an herbalist, a nutritionist, *and* a Victoria's Secret model—so we kind of (definitely) get her early exposure to healthy foods and her ability to capture an audience. With four cookbooks, Rens has developed what she calls a "powerfood" lifestyle (as in, focusing on highly nutritious and unprocessed food)—and this recipe is one of her go-tos. She often makes an extra-big batch to enjoy as leftovers the next day. "I secretly think it's even tastier when it's had a bit of time to sit," she adds.

TEMPEH TIKKA MASALA

Serves 4 to 6

⅔ cup bulgur

1½ cups boiling water

3½ ounces unsalted raw cashews, soaked in water for at least 30 minutes or up to overnight and drained

8 ounces tempeh, cut into ¼-inch cubes

3 tablespoons ghee or coconut oil, melted

½ teaspoon smoked paprika

2 small red onions, diced

3 garlic cloves, minced

¼ to ½ teaspoon chili powder

½ teaspoon garam masala

1 (14.5-ounce) can crushed tomatoes

1 teaspoon sea salt

Freshly ground black pepper

Handful of fresh cilantro, finely chopped, for serving

VEGAN

VEGETARIAN

BETTER FOCUS

1. Place the bulgur in a small bowl and pour over the boiling water. Cover and let stand for 10 minutes. Drain the excess water and cover again to keep the bulgur warm.

2. In a high-speed blender or food processor, combine the soaked cashews and ½ cup water. Blend until completely smooth. Set the cashew cream aside.

3. Brush the tempeh all over with 1 tablespoon of the melted ghee and season with the paprika.

4. Heat the remaining 2 tablespoons ghee in a large skillet over medium-high heat. When it shimmers, add the onions and cook, stirring, until translucent, about 3 minutes. Add the tempeh, garlic, chili powder (use more or less to taste), and garam masala and cook, stirring often, for 1 to 2 minutes, until warm. Add the tomatoes, salt, and cashew cream and season with pepper. Stir well to combine and warm through, 2 to 3 minutes.

5. Transfer the bulgur to a serving dish. Layer the tempeh-tomato mixture on top. Sprinkle with the cilantro and serve.

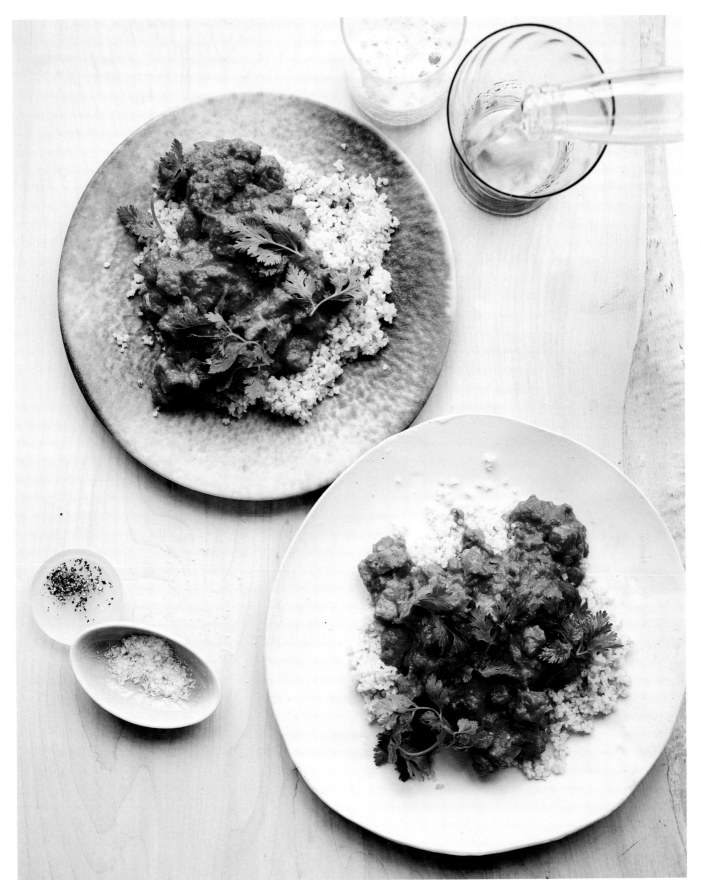

SWEETS
+ SNACKS

Frank Lipman, MD, is a trailblazer in the world of functional and integrative medicine, but his wife, Janice, was super ahead of her husband's cravings curve with this nondairy dessert. "I love ice cream, but not the sugar, so my wife helped me create this recipe so I could indulge," says the founder of Be Well, an expanding lifestyle wellness brand. This frosty treat (guaranteed to be your new obsession) only takes a few minutes if you plan ahead and refrigerate the coconut milk overnight.

CHOCOLATE ICE CREAM

Serves 2

1 (13.5-ounce) can full-fat coconut milk, refrigerated overnight

1 tablespoon chocolate whey protein powder

1 teaspoon raw cacao powder

1 tablespoon smooth almond butter

8 to 10 ice cubes

1. Open the can of chilled coconut milk and scoop the solid white cream into a high-speed blender, reserving the clear liquid underneath. Add the protein powder, cacao powder, almond butter, ice, and 2 to 3 tablespoons of the reserved coconut liquid. Blend, gradually increasing the speed from low to high, until completely smooth. Add more of the reserved coconut liquid as needed until the desired consistency is reached.

2. Divide the ice cream between two bowls and enjoy immediately.

Tip: Save the remaining liquid from the can of coconut milk to use in smoothies.

GLUTEN-FREE

VEGETARIAN

BETTER ENERGY

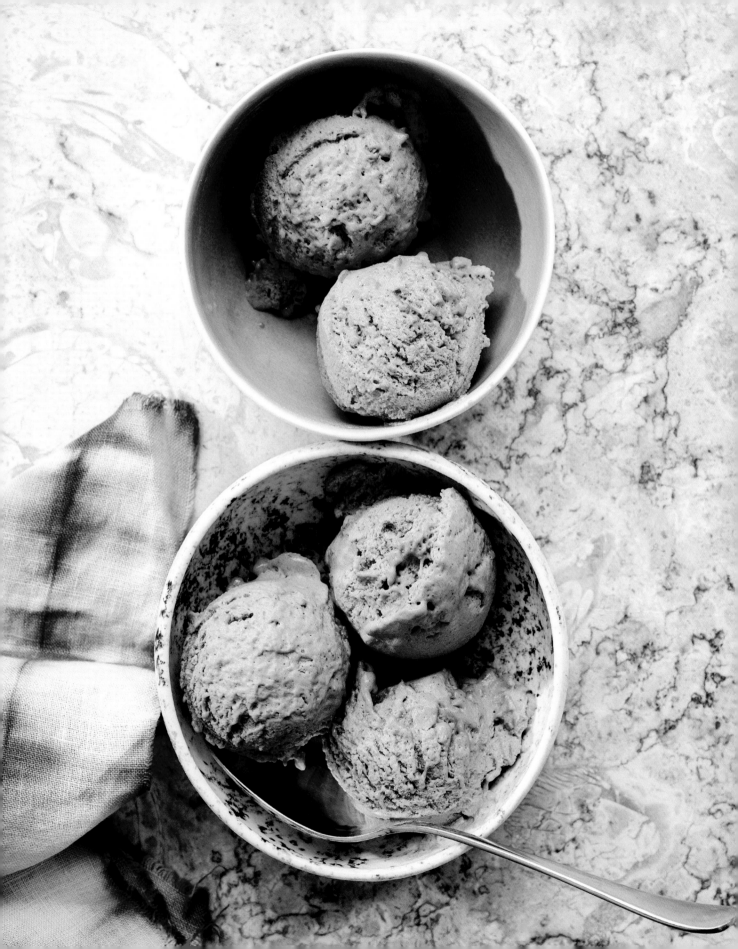

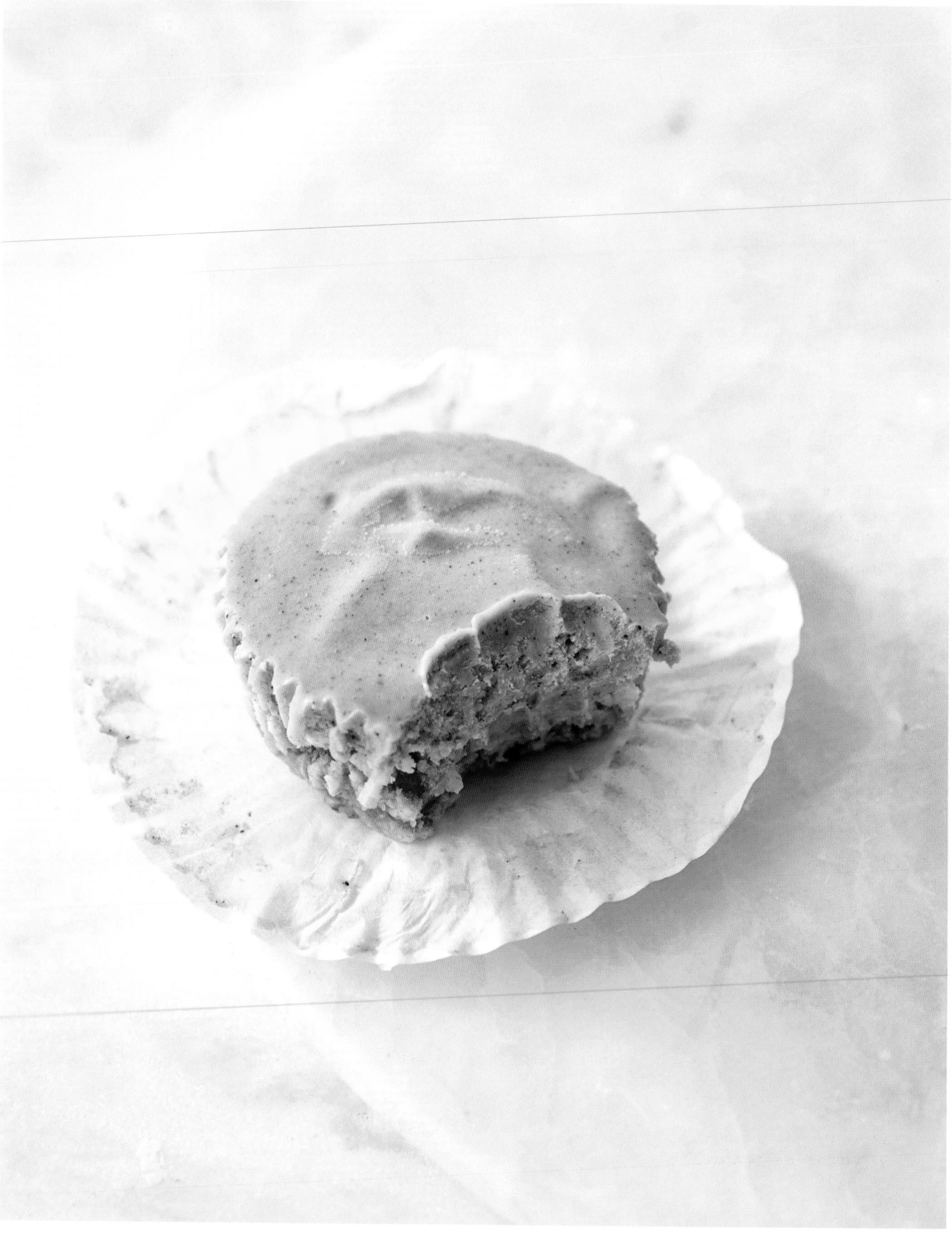

"Cooking should be colorful, not complicated," says health coach and food blogger Ilene Godofsky Moreno. The author of *The Colorful Kitchen* cookbook has a penchant for easy, plant-based recipes that look as good as they taste—even if you don't have her food photography skills. These superfood sweets don't require any baking, giving raw-food power to the people after only a few hours of cooling in the fridge.

MINI GOLDEN MILK CREAM CUPS

Makes 20 mini cups

FOR THE CRUST

¼ cup pitted dates, such as Medjool or Deglet Noor

¾ cup rolled oats

¼ cup unsweetened shredded coconut

2 tablespoons coconut oil, melted

1 tablespoon pure maple syrup

Pinch of sea salt

FOR THE GOLDEN MILK CREAM

1 cup raw cashews, soaked in water for at least 4 hours or overnight, and drained

1 (13.5-ounce) can full-fat coconut milk, refrigerated overnight

1 tablespoon pure maple syrup

1 tablespoon coconut oil, melted

½ teaspoon pure vanilla extract

1 tablespoon ground turmeric

1 teaspoon ground cinnamon

¼ teaspoon kosher salt

2 tablespoons coconut butter, melted, for drizzling (optional)

1. Make the crust. Line two mini-muffin tins with paper liners.

2. If the dates are not already soft, put them in a bowl and add hot water to cover. Set aside to soak for 30 minutes, then drain.

3. In a blender or food processor, pulse the oats until a flour forms. Add the dates, shredded coconut, coconut oil, maple syrup, and salt and pulse until the ingredients are well incorporated and the texture is mostly smooth. Scoop slightly less than 1 tablespoon into each prepared muffin cup and use your fingers to press it firmly into the bottoms of the cups.

4. Make the golden milk cream. Place the cashews in the blender. Open the can of chilled coconut milk and scoop the thick white cream into the blender, reserving the clear liquid underneath. Add 2 tablespoons of the reserved coconut liquid, the maple syrup, coconut oil, vanilla, turmeric, cinnamon, and salt. Blend until completely smooth, scraping the sides down as needed to fully incorporate.

5. Pour the golden milk cream into the prepared muffin cups over the crust. Refrigerate for at least 1 hour or overnight, until the cups are firm to the touch.

6. Remove the cups from the muffin tin, peel off the liners, and set the cups on a baking sheet or platter. Use a spoon to drizzle the melted coconut butter over the tops. Return the cups to the refrigerator for at least 20 minutes to set.

7. Enjoy, or store in an airtight container in the refrigerator for up to 1 week.

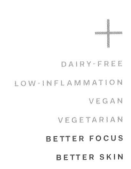

DAIRY-FREE

LOW-INFLAMMATION

VEGAN

VEGETARIAN

BETTER FOCUS

BETTER SKIN

Well+Good Council member Gabrielle Bernstein—who also has the Oprah stamp of approval as a "next-generation thought leader"—credits this fudge (and the guidance of her nutritionist, Cat Marcellino) with saving her from sugar cravings by giving her extra energy and fueling her brain with healthy fats like ghee and coconut oil. "It helps me stick to my no-sugar, high-protein and -fat diet, which aids my digestion and gut health," says the six-time modern spirituality author. This mind-boost is a no-brainer—and you can totally pop it in the freezer and eat it straight out of the bowl if you don't feel like forming full-on fudge squares.

SUGAR-FREE TAHINI FUDGE

Makes 4 squares

1 tablespoon ghee

2 tablespoons coconut oil

3 tablespoons tahini

2 teaspoons pure vanilla extract

Pinch of sea salt

Ground cinnamon

1. Line a 4-inch square baking dish with parchment paper, leaving a 2-inch overhang on all four sides.

2. In a medium bowl, combine the ghee, coconut oil, tahini, vanilla, salt, and cinnamon to taste. Using a spatula, mix well until the ingredients are thoroughly combined.

3. Pour the mixture into the prepared pan and freeze for at least 30 minutes or overnight, until the fudge is hardened. Using the overhanging parchment as handles, remove the block from the pan and cut it into four 2-inch squares.

4. Store in a freezer-safe container in the freezer for up to 1 month.

GLUTEN-FREE

KETOGENIC

LOW-INFLAMMATION

PALEO

VEGETARIAN

BETTER DIGESTION

BETTER ENERGY

BETTER FOCUS

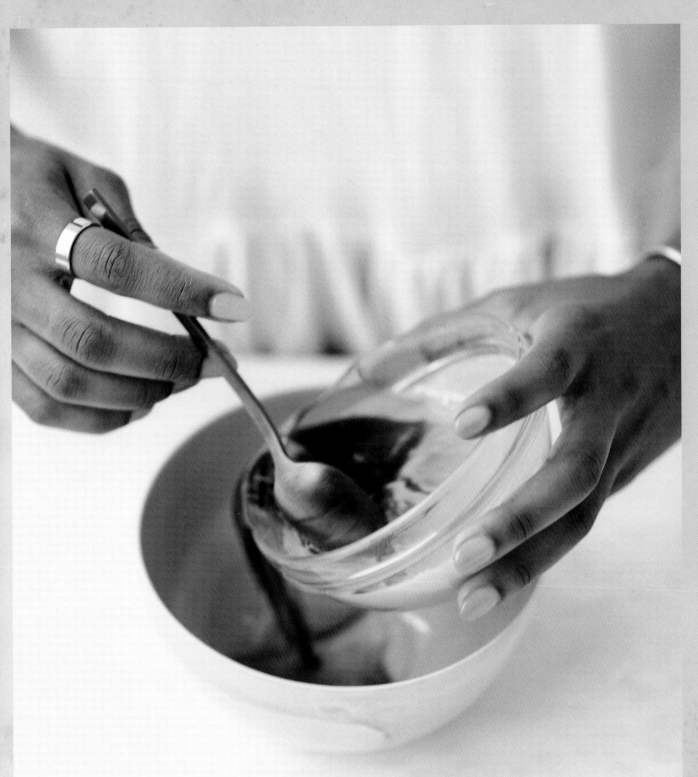

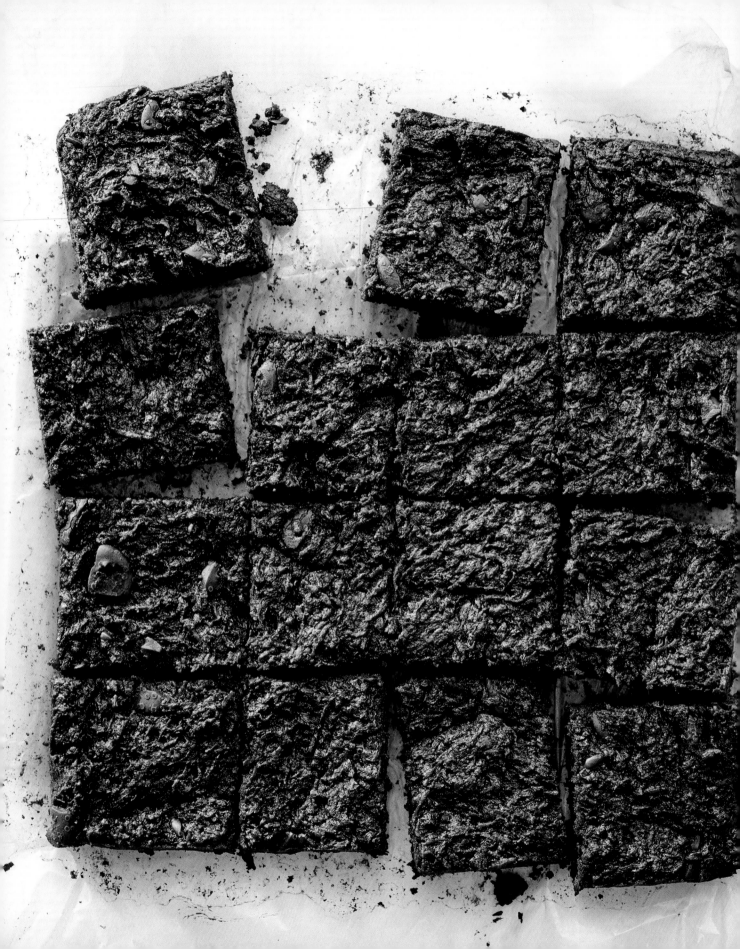

Known as the "hormone whisperer," functional nutrition expert and founder of FLO Living Hormone Center, Alisa Vitti, HHC, shares easy brownies she created to relieve some major symptoms of PMS, which she believes is largely treatable with food. Alisa says cacao, sweet potatoes, almond butter, and flaxseed can help increase progesterone, stabilize blood sugar, and balance estrogen levels—which alleviates breast tenderness and combats bloating. Toss a few extra chocolate chips into the batter for extra brownie points—just saying.

PMS-BUSTING BROWNIES

Makes 16 brownies

2 tablespoons ground flaxseed

1 medium Japanese sweet potato, finely grated (about 2½ cups)

¼ cup honey, coconut nectar, or pure maple syrup

1 teaspoon pure vanilla extract

½ cup coconut oil, melted

½ cup raw cacao powder

1 teaspoon ground cinnamon

1 teaspoon baking powder

1 teaspoon baking soda

2 tablespoons coconut flour, teff flour, buckwheat flour, or oat flour

2 tablespoons arrowroot powder

¼ teaspoon pink Himalayan salt

½ cup chocolate chips (optional)

Raspberries or strawberries and coconut yogurt, for serving

1. Preheat the oven to 375°F. Line a 9-inch square baking dish with parchment paper, leaving a 2-inch overhang on two sides.

2. In a medium bowl, mix together the flaxseed and ¼ cup water. Add the sweet potato, honey, vanilla, and coconut oil. Stir until well incorporated.

3. In a separate medium bowl, combine the cacao powder, cinnamon, baking powder, baking soda, flour, arrowroot, and salt.

4. Add the wet ingredients to the dry ingredients and mix well. Fold in the chocolate chips. Pour the batter into the prepared pan and smooth the top with a spatula.

5. Bake for 25 to 30 minutes, until a tester inserted into the center comes out clean. Let cool in the pan for 10 minutes, then use the overhanging parchment as handles and remove the brownie block from the pan. Cut the block into 16 squares (4 rows by 4 rows).

6. Serve with fruit and coconut yogurt for extra decadence. Store in an airtight container at room temperature for up to 3 days or wrapped in plastic wrap in the freezer for up to 3 months.

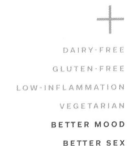

DAIRY-FREE

GLUTEN-FREE

LOW-INFLAMMATION

VEGETARIAN

BETTER MOOD

BETTER SEX

This sugar-free dessert came to life based on fitness foodie Crosby Tailor's nostalgia for the York Peppermint Patties that were always abundant at his grandparents' house. "My goal in this world of sweets is to take all my favorite indulgences and turn them into healthy—yet delicious—desserts," says the personal trainer and founder of Crosby's Cookies, a sugar-free, gluten-free, and grain-free dessert company. Here he hacks the original by removing the sugar and adding nutrient-packed superfoods and MCT oil, the metabolism-revving fats found in coconuts. Don't have a silicone tray? A repurposed ice cube tray will do the trick if you're careful about popping them out.

MINT CHOCOLATE SUPERFOOD SQUARES

Makes 8 squares

¼ cup plus 1 tablespoon monk fruit sweetener

3 tablespoons cacao butter

½ cup raw cacao powder

3 pinches of pink Himalayan salt

4 tablespoons MCT oil

8 drops of vanilla-flavored liquid stevia

1 tablespoon collagen powder

½ teaspoon greens powder

Peppermint spirits (12 to 20 drops) to taste

1. In a food processor or blender, or using a mortar and pestle, grind the monk fruit sweetener into a fine powder.

2. Melt the cacao butter in a small saucepan over low heat. Remove the pan from the heat and let the cacao butter cool slightly.

3. In a medium bowl, whisk together the cacao powder, ¼ cup of the monk fruit sweetener, and 2 pinches of the salt. Slowly whisk in 2 tablespoons of the melted cacao butter, 3 tablespoons of the MCT oil, and the stevia until smooth. Fill about 8 slots in a silicone tray with 1½ teaspoons of the chocolate mixture. Freeze for 5 to 10 minutes, until hardened.

4. Meanwhile, in a separate medium bowl, whisk together the collagen powder, greens powder, and remaining 1 tablespoon monk fruit sweetener. Slowly whisk in the remaining 1 tablespoon melted cacao butter and 1 tablespoon MCT oil. Add peppermint spirits to taste and whisk until smooth.

5. Remove the hardened chocolate from the freezer. Spread ½ teaspoon of the peppermint mixture onto the top of the chocolate to create the centers. Shake the tray to evenly distribute the mint layer. Freeze for 5 to 10 minutes, until hardened.

6. Remove from the freezer again and add another layer of chocolate, about 1½ teaspoons, to each. Freeze for at least 25 minutes more or overnight, until completely hardened and easy to remove from the tray.

7. Store in a freezer-safe airtight container in the freezer for up to 2 weeks.

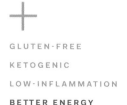

GLUTEN-FREE

KETOGENIC

LOW-INFLAMMATION

BETTER ENERGY

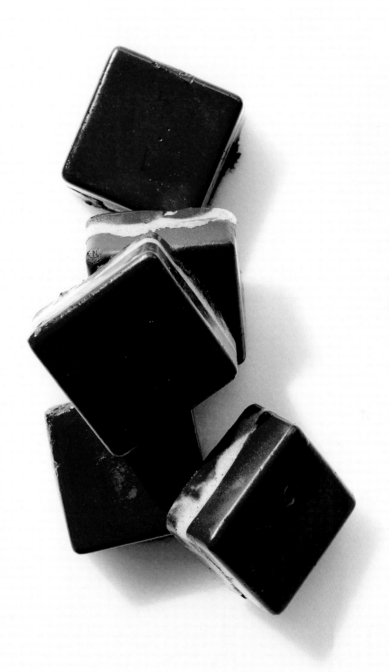

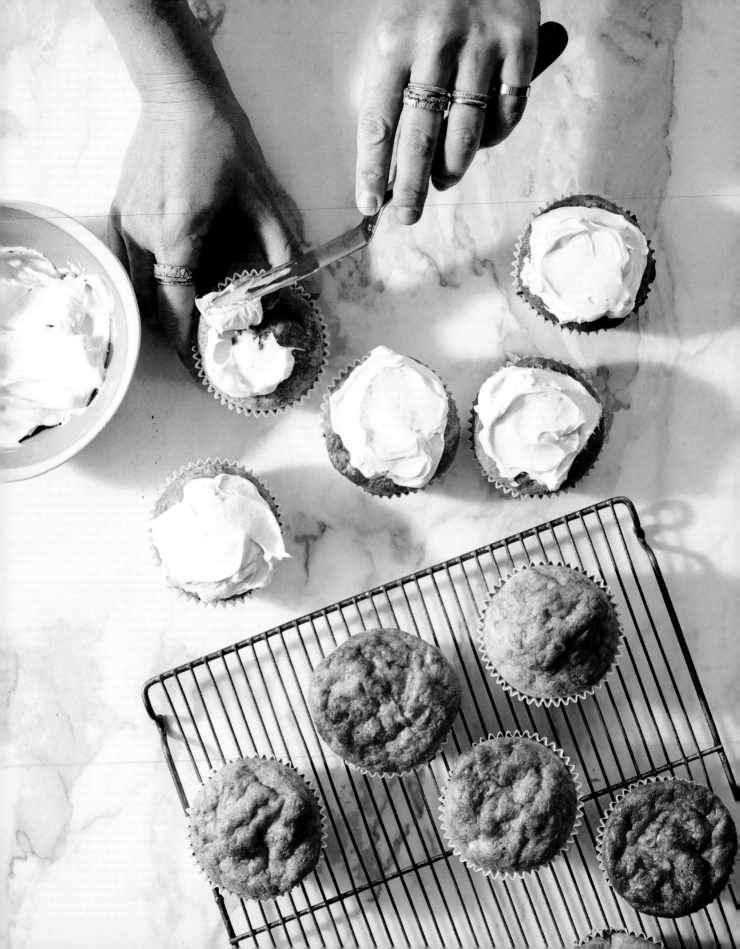

As a mom, Tanya Zuckerbrot—a New York City–based registered dietitian and author of *The F-Factor Diet*—always has baby carrots on hand and in her fridge, so she devised a delicious way to use the dregs of any given bag. "This dessert is so easy to whip up and keeps the carrots from going to waste," she says. Carrots contain her all-time favorite nutrient (F-Factor = fiber!), which can help sustain energy, clear skin, and combat bloating. After putting the cupcakes in the oven, don't ignore the temperature switch—the initial high heat activates the baking powder, giving the cupcakes a fluffy consistency, while the remaining time and lower temp bakes them through.

CARROT CUPCAKES

Makes 16 cupcakes

FOR THE CUPCAKES

Coconut oil cooking spray

7 egg whites

1 large egg

1 tablespoon coconut oil

½ cup nonfat Greek yogurt

½ teaspoon pure vanilla extract

1 cup vanilla protein powder

3 tablespoons all-natural erythritol brown sugar alternative

½ cup almond flour

1 teaspoon baking powder

½ teaspoon baking soda

2 cups freshly shredded carrots

½ teaspoon freshly grated nutmeg

1 teaspoon ground cinnamon

FOR THE FROSTING

8 ounces Greek cream cheese

1 teaspoon pure vanilla extract

1 tablespoon vanilla protein powder

1. Preheat the oven to 425°F. Line two 12-cup muffin tins with paper liners and spray with the cooking spray.

2. Make the cupcakes. In a large bowl, whisk together the egg whites, egg, coconut oil, and Greek yogurt until smooth. Add the vanilla, protein powder, brown sugar alternative, almond flour, baking powder, baking soda, carrots, nutmeg, and cinnamon and mix until completely smooth.

3. Spoon the batter into the prepared muffin tins, filling each cup about three-quarters of the way. Bake for 10 minutes, then reduce the oven temperature to 350°F. Bake for 20 to 25 minutes more, until a tester inserted into the center of a cupcake comes out clean.

4. Remove the muffin tins from the oven. Let the cupcakes cool in the pans for 5 to 7 minutes, then transfer them to a wire rack and allow them to cool completely.

5. While the cupcakes cool, make the frosting. In a medium bowl, combine the cream cheese and vanilla extract. Using a spatula, mix thoroughly. Slowly stir in the protein powder, a little bit at a time, and stir until fully incorporated.

6. Frost the cooled cupcakes as desired and enjoy. Store in an airtight container at room temperature for 2 to 3 days.

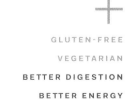

GLUTEN-FREE

VEGETARIAN

BETTER DIGESTION

BETTER ENERGY

Kelsey Patel is one of Los Angeles's most sought-after wellness experts—but you could say the MVP of this recipe is actually her husband, Ap. "Since I was a little girl, I've loved Reese's Peanut Butter Cups," explains the spiritual empowerment coach and Reiki-trained meditation teacher. "So when I'd go on work trips, my husband would buy a pack of them and stick it in my suitcase as a surprise for me to find later." But as Kelsey started paying more attention to what was in her food, she realized she needed a better solution to quell her chocolate-peanut butter craving. Her personal chef, Leigh, helped develop these no-bakes to perfectly complement the couple's balanced approach to food, which mostly includes organic veggies, healthy grains, and clean proteins, but still allows for the occasional takeout pizza and red wine.

PEANUT BUTTER CUPS

Makes 12 peanut butter cups

¾ cup peanut butter

1 tablespoon pure maple syrup

½ cup coconut oil, melted

½ cup unsweetened cocoa powder

3 tablespoons honey

Coarse sea salt

1. Line a mini-muffin tin with paper liners.

2. In a small bowl, stir together the peanut butter and maple syrup. Place 1 heaping tablespoon of the mixture in each prepared muffin cup. Freeze for at least 30 minutes or overnight, until hardened.

3. In a medium bowl, whisk together the coconut oil, cocoa powder, and honey until smooth and glossy.

4. Pour 1 tablespoon of the chocolate glaze on top of each hardened peanut butter cup and sprinkle with a pinch of sea salt. Freeze for at least 20 minutes, or until the glaze hardens, before serving.

5. Store in an airtight container in the freezer for up to 2 weeks.

DAIRY-FREE

GLUTEN-FREE

VEGETARIAN

BETTER ENERGY

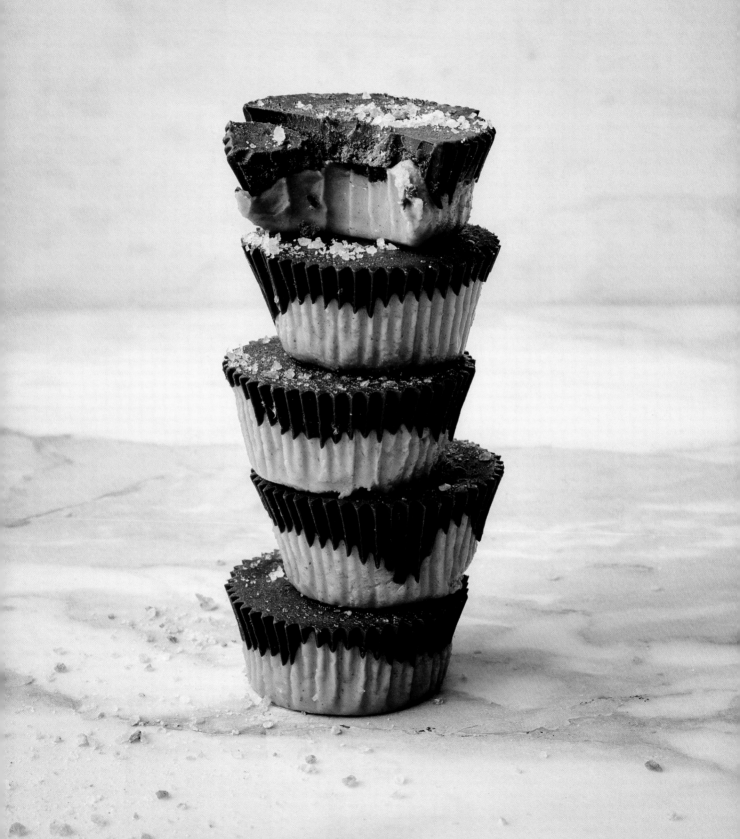

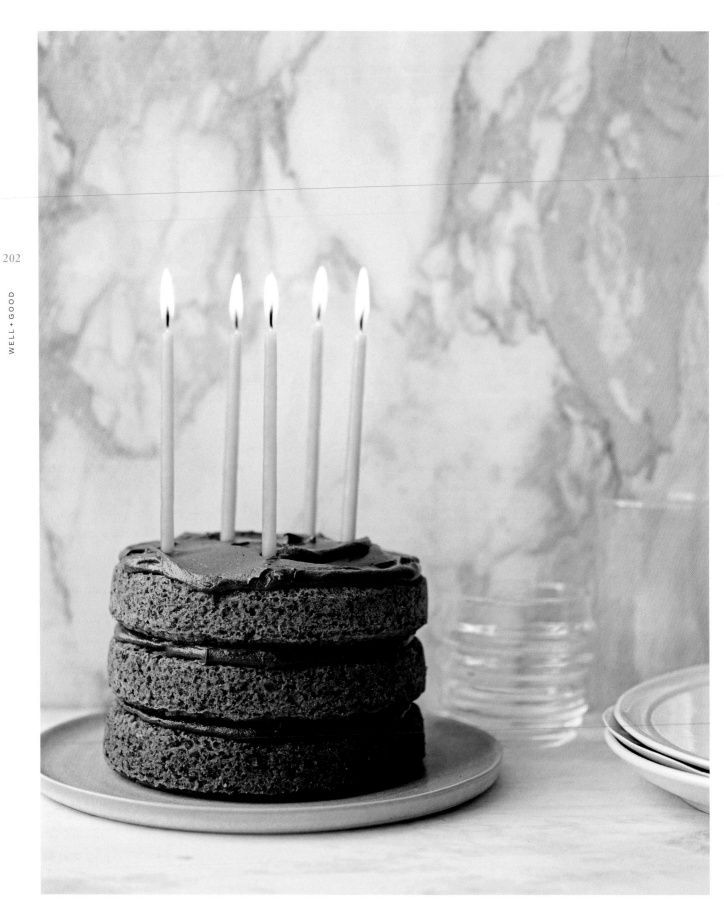

When Hashimoto's disease left Laurel Gallucci with digestive dysfunction (aka an inability to digest food properly) and secondary amenorrhea (meaning without periods), her doctor challenged her to remove all grains, legumes, and refined sugar from her diet. "I saw incredible leaps in my health," says the founder (with Claire Thomas) of whole foods bakery Sweet Laurel and coauthor of the cookbook of the same name. "We have many customers who take their healing to the next level with the ketogenic diet," she says, which led her to craft this seriously celebration-worthy dessert. Now you can have your keto cake and eat it, too.

KETO BIRTHDAY CAKE

Makes one 6-inch cake

FOR THE CAKE

1 tablespoon coconut oil

3 cups almond meal or almond flour

2 tablespoons coconut flour

1 teaspoon baking soda

1 teaspoon ground turmeric

1 teaspoon pink Himalayan salt

¾ cup monk fruit sweetener

3 large eggs

1½ tablespoons pure vanilla extract

FOR THE GANACHE

4 tablespoons coconut oil

4 ounces unsweetened baking chocolate (100% cacao)

3 tablespoons monk fruit sweetener

1 cup coconut milk, plus more if needed

1. Make the cake. Preheat the oven to 350°F. Grease three 6-inch cake pans with the coconut oil, then line them with parchment paper cut to fit.

2. In a medium bowl, stir together the almond meal, coconut flour, baking soda, turmeric, salt, and monk fruit. Add the eggs, vanilla, and ¾ cup water and mix well to combine.

3. Divide the batter evenly among the prepared pans and smooth the tops. Bake for 25 minutes, or until a tester inserted into the center of one cake comes out clean. Let cool completely in the pans.

4. Meanwhile, make the ganache. In a medium pan, combine the coconut oil and baking chocolate and melt over low heat, stirring. Remove the pan from the heat and, while whisking, slowly add the monk fruit, then the coconut milk. Whisk until completely smooth, adding more coconut milk or water as needed to reach the desired consistency. Let cool completely.

5. Assemble the cake. Place one cake layer on a cake plate and top with 2 to 3 tablespoons of the ganache and spread evenly to the edges. Repeat with the remaining cake layers and ganache. Keep at room temperature until ready to enjoy.

+

DAIRY-FREE

GLUTEN-FREE

KETOGENIC

LOW-INFLAMMATION

VEGETARIAN

BETTER MOOD

Traveling full-time with international pop star Tove Lo means a lot of road snacks for Courtney Swan, an integrative nutritionist and food activist. And as any road warrior knows, sometimes you have to improvise—and that's how these kombucha gummies were born. "I am always looking for ways to make my favorite treats healthier," says the *Realfoodology* blogger. Invest in a tray mold to make these gummies, which are a fun way to ingest your probiotics on the go, whether you're on a tour bus, in an airport, or just dashing from meetings to the gym. A word of caution: Don't let the mixture boil or get too hot, or you will kill off the beneficial bacteria!

PICK-YOUR-FAVORITE
KOMBUCHA GUMMIES

*Makes 8 to 12 large gummies
or 100 gummy bears*

1 cup unsweetened coconut water

½ cup unsweetened grass-fed gelatin powder

1 cup kombucha

1 (1-inch) piece fresh ginger, peeled and puréed (see Tip, page 226)

1 teaspoon pure maple syrup or coconut sugar (or more for sweeter gummies)

½ cup fresh lemon juice (from 2 or 3 lemons)

Silicone molds

1. Bring the coconut water to a simmer in a medium saucepan over low heat, about 10 minutes.

2. Meanwhile, place the gelatin in a small bowl and pour over the kombucha. Whisk to combine, then set aside to bloom for 5 minutes.

3. Remove the pan from the heat. Add the gelatin mixture, ginger, maple syrup, and lemon juice and whisk to combine. Return the pan to medium heat and bring to a simmer, then cook, whisking often, until the gelatin has fully dissolved, about 5 minutes.

4. Pour the mixture into the silicone molds. Refrigerate for at least 1 hour 30 minutes, until hard. Store the gummies in an airtight container in the refrigerator for about 1 week.

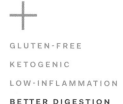

GLUTEN-FREE

KETOGENIC

LOW-INFLAMMATION

BETTER DIGESTION

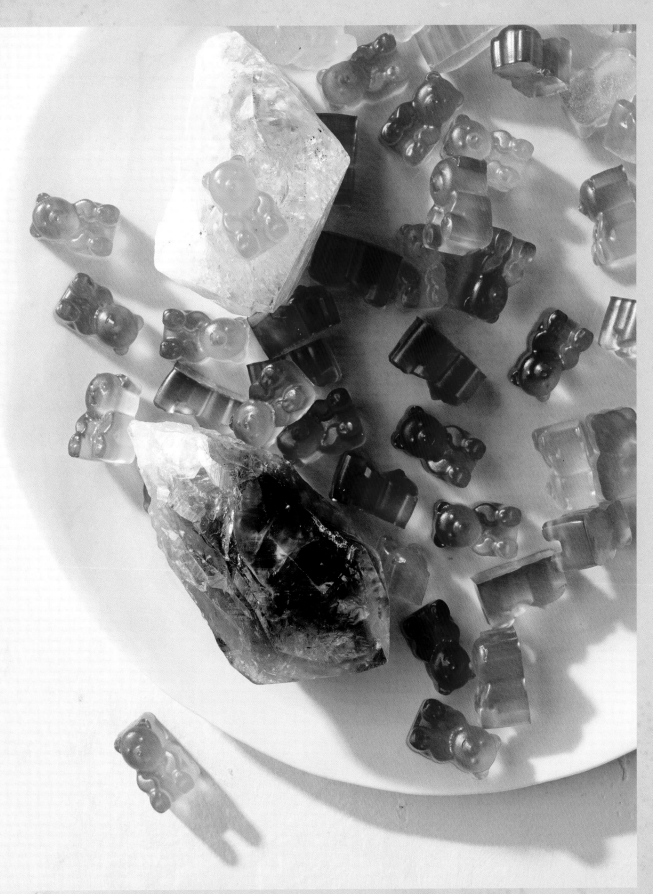

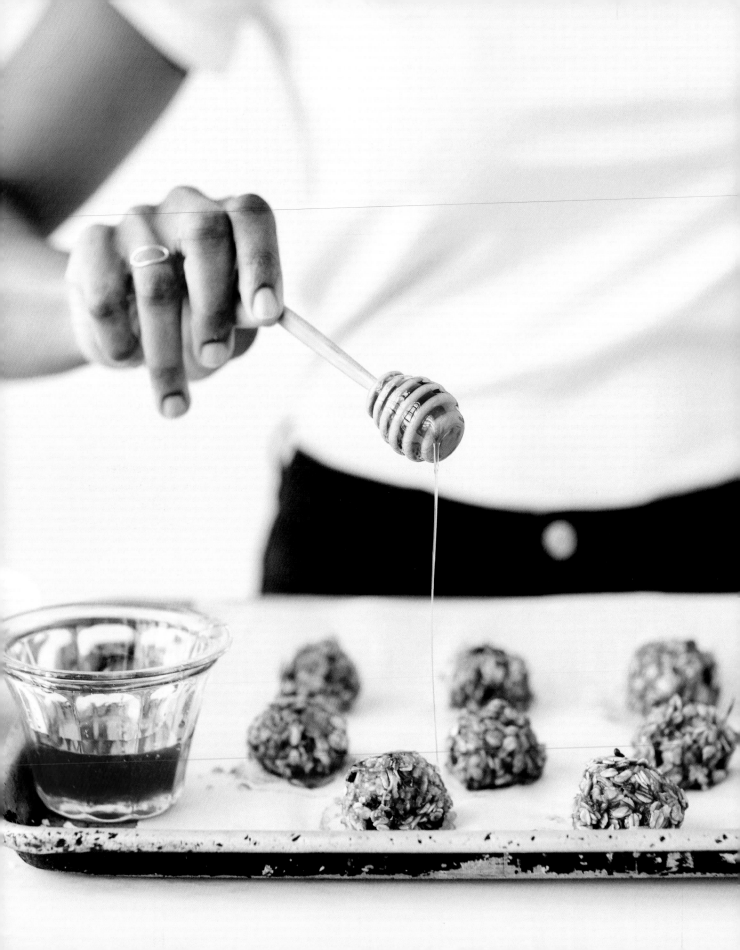

JORDANA
KIER

+

ALEXANDRA
FRIEDMAN

"We think wellness is all about balance—not just for your body—but your mind also," say fem-tech entrepreneurs Jordana Kier and Alexandra Friedman. The duo founded Lola, a brand focused on organic products for women's reproductive health and wellness, for everything from periods to sex. Their company is based on transparency—and that includes being honest with *themselves*, as in admitting when a sweet tooth can't just be ignored. Jordana and Alexandra enjoy these secret weapons of tastiness whenever they feel an urge to fill up on junk food. And good news: A well-stocked pantry means you probably already have these ingredients on hand.

PEANUT BUTTER–BANANA BALLS

Makes 8 to 10 balls

2 ripe medium bananas, mashed

¼ cup unsweetened shredded coconut, plus more for topping

2 teaspoons cacao nibs

1 cup rolled oats

2 tablespoons smooth peanut butter

Sea salt

Drizzle of honey (optional)

1. Preheat the oven to 325°F. Line a baking sheet with parchment paper.

2. In a medium bowl, stir together the bananas, shredded coconut, cacao nibs, oats, and peanut butter with a spatula until a moist dough forms. With clean hands, form the mixture into 1-inch balls and place them on the prepared baking sheet. Sprinkle a light pinch of salt over the tops.

3. Bake for 15 minutes, or until a toothpick inserted into the center of a ball comes out clean. Remove from the oven and let cool for about 15 minutes. Drizzle honey over the balls, if desired, and sprinkle with more shredded coconut. Refrigerate for at least 20 minutes or overnight, until hardened.

4. Store in an airtight container in the refrigerator for up to 2 weeks.

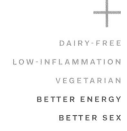

DAIRY-FREE

LOW-INFLAMMATION

VEGETARIAN

BETTER ENERGY

BETTER SEX

EAT FOR BETTER SEX

Some foods are just sexier than others. Oysters, figs, asparagus, and chocolate, for example, have long been viewed as aphrodisiacs because of how sensual they look or how we feel when we eat them. And, in each case, science can explain how they've earned their reputation as libido-boosters.

Oysters are packed with amino acids and zinc, both of which increase reproductive hormones and support sexual stamina. Figs are high in zinc, too, along with magnesium, two minerals that, together, boost testosterone and other sex hormones. Asparagus doesn't just look phallic; it also contains B vitamins and potassium, both of which increase arousal and enhance orgasm. And chocolate definitely deserves its association with sexual pleasure, thanks to phenethylamine (PEA for short), which promotes the production of dopamine, a neurotransmitter that increases our sense of well-being and capacity for pleasure.

We shouldn't neglect foods that put out a less sexy image, though. Celery, for example, contains plant steroids that can have a subtle positive effect on the pheromones our bodies release to attract the opposite sex.

Speaking of odors, garlic may be pungent, but don't let that put you off. Thanks to a compound called allicin, it has a measurable effect on blood flow, which leads to better bedroom endurance and more sensation. (Just make sure you keep the breath mints handy!)

And while high-fiber foods, such as beans and legumes, may have a reputation for giving people gas, they also benefit intestinal health, and in doing so, they have a positive effect on hormone balance.

SCIENCE CAN EXPLAIN
HOW MANY FOODS
HAVE EARNED THEIR
REPUTATIONS AS
LIBIDO-BOOSTERS.

It's important to remember, though, that a food's ability to enhance our sex lives isn't just about its nutritional components—it's also the result of how it makes us feel. After all, in many ancient cultures, sex was seen as an energetic exchange where both partners give and receive pleasure. When this energy is powerful and flows freely, the result is connected, meaningful sex.

Here are the lesser-known healthy foods that, according to Traditional Chinese Medicine and modern nutritional science, can add to your sexual well-being and experience:

FOODS THAT HELP YOU GIVE PLEASURE BY OFFERING ENERGY. Choose warming, tonifying foods including carrots, parsnips, mushrooms, sweet potatoes, squash, chiles, ginger, beans, walnuts, lamb, and salmon.

FOODS THAT HELP YOU RECEIVE PLEASURE BY PROVIDING NOURISHMENT. Choose foods with high water content and nutrient density, including seaweed, beets, flaxseeds, spinach, chard, cucumbers, string beans, grapes, watermelon, millet, amaranth, eggs, mung beans, nuts, and sunflower seeds.

FOODS THAT HELP INCREASE SENSATION BY PROMOTING CIRCULATION. These foods include broccoli, kohlrabi, turnips, cauliflower, peppermint, radish, parsley, tomato, celery, asparagus, oranges, lemons, strawberries, buckwheat, sesame seeds, lima beans, fish, fava beans, chia seeds, pistachios, and yogurt.

—JILL BLAKEWAY,
LAC, DACM

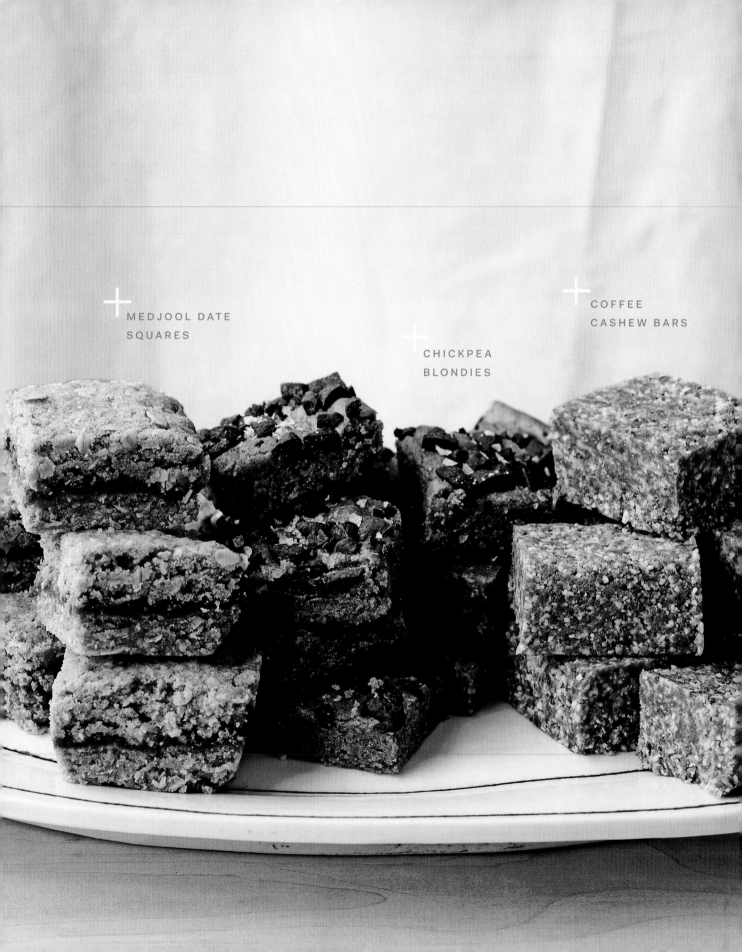

+ MEDJOOL DATE
SQUARES

+ CHICKPEA
BLONDIES

+ COFFEE
CASHEW BARS

CHLOE COSCARELLI

If there's one ingredient that's completely underestimated, in Chloe Coscarelli's opinion, it's dates. "These little gems are packed with vitamins and minerals and bursting with sticky, caramel-y sweetness—reminding me that our universe is truly magical," says the trendsetting vegan chef, restaurateur, and four-time cookbook author (who's pretty darn magical herself). Chloe often makes these treats for friends, who almost always ask for the recipe after just a few bites. Be prepared to fill your home with a warm cinnamon-oat scent as they bake—another added benefit of nature's natural sweetener.

MEDJOOL DATE SQUARES

Makes sixteen 2-inch squares

FOR THE CRUMB MIXTURE

1½ cups all-purpose flour

1 cup packed brown sugar

2 teaspoons ground cinnamon

½ teaspoon baking soda

½ teaspoon kosher salt

1 cup vegan margarine (plus a little extra to grease the pan)

1 cup rolled oats

FOR THE FILLING

1 cup pitted dates, such as Medjool or Deglet Noor

2 teaspoons pure vanilla extract

Confectioners' sugar, for dusting (optional)

1. Preheat the oven to 350°F. Lightly grease an 8-inch square pan and line it with parchment paper, leaving a 2-inch overhang on all sides.

2. Make the crumb mixture. In a food processor, combine the flour, brown sugar, cinnamon, baking soda, and salt. Process until completely combined. Add the margarine and the oats, and process until the mixture is combined but still coarse.

3. Make the filling. In a small pot, combine the dates and 1 cup water. Bring the water to a boil over high heat and cook for about 10 minutes, until the water has been almost completely absorbed. Transfer the dates and any liquid remaining in the pot to a food processor and add the vanilla. Process until almost smooth, adding an additional 1 tablespoon water as needed until the mixture reaches the desired consistency. Transfer the filling to a medium bowl and let cool.

4. Transfer two-thirds of the crumb mixture to the prepared pan and press it down firmly using your fingers or the bottom of a measuring cup. Spread the date filling evenly over the top. Sprinkle the remaining crumb mixture all over. Bake for 40 minutes, or until lightly browned.

5. Remove from the oven and let cool completely in the pan. Using the overhanging parchment as handles, remove the block from the pan and cut it into 2-inch squares.

6. Dust the squares with confectioners' sugar, if desired. Store in an airtight container in the refrigerator for up to 1 week.

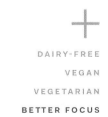

DAIRY-FREE

VEGAN

VEGETARIAN

BETTER FOCUS

Yes, you can have a little something sweet after dinner without detonating a sugar bomb, says celebrity nutritionist Molly Rieger. Molly, who curated the dairy-free menu at the beach-themed healthy eatery Broken Coconut in New York City, sneakily uses chickpeas in this batter (you can't even taste them!), which ramp up the protein and fiber content. "These blondies will leave you feeling empowered rather than deprived," she says. "Focus on all the amazing whole, natural, delicious foods you get to nourish your body with, rather than what you 'can't' or 'shouldn't' eat."

CHICKPEA BLONDIES

Makes 16 blondies

Coconut oil spray

1 (15-ounce) can chickpeas, drained and rinsed

½ cup almond butter or peanut butter

⅓ cup pure maple syrup or honey

2 teaspoons pure vanilla extract

½ teaspoon sea salt, plus more as needed

¼ teaspoon baking powder

¼ teaspoon baking soda

⅓ cup dark vegan chocolate chips

1. Preheat the oven to 350°F. Coat an 8-inch square pan with coconut oil spray.

2. In a blender or food processor, combine the chickpeas, almond butter, maple syrup, vanilla, salt, baking powder, and baking soda. Process until completely smooth. Transfer the batter to the prepared pan and use a spatula to spread it evenly and smooth out the top. Scatter the chocolate chips on top.

3. Bake for 20 to 25 minutes, until a tester inserted into the center comes out clean. Remove the pan from the oven and set it on a wire rack. Let the blondies cool for 20 minutes, then sprinkle with a pinch of sea salt and cut into 2-inch squares.

4. Store in an airtight container at room temperature for up to 1 week or wrapped in plastic in the freezer for up to 3 months.

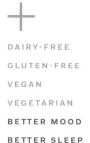

DAIRY-FREE

GLUTEN-FREE

VEGAN

VEGETARIAN

BETTER MOOD

BETTER SLEEP

"I love creating food that's accessible and enjoyable for everyone, from the kitchen expert to someone who is just starting out making healthier food and lifestyle changes," says Mia Zarlengo, MS, RD, recipe developer, and blogger behind *Bites by Mia*. She came up with the concept for these afternoon pick-me-ups along her path to healing her chronic fatigue, acid reflux, and autoimmune condition (Hashimoto's disease), all while studying for her master's degree in nutrition. True to her philosophy, this snack is easy to whip up. Plus, it's low in sugar, with lots of healthy fat—and it *contains coffee*. Put down the extra cup. Your afternoon snack: solved.

COFFEE CASHEW BARS

Makes 16 bars

1½ cups raw cashews

½ cup unsweetened shredded coconut

¼ cup coconut flour

3 pitted dates, such as Medjool or Deglet Noor, quartered

1 tablespoon chia seeds

1 tablespoon brewed room-temperature coffee (or more, for a stronger coffee flavor)

1 tablespoon almond milk or coconut milk

1 teaspoon pure vanilla extract

1 teaspoon pure maple syrup

1 teaspoon unsweetened cocoa powder

1 teaspoon ground cinnamon

1 teaspoon MCT oil or melted coconut oil

1. Line an 8 by 8-inch loaf pan with parchment paper, leaving a 2-inch overhang on all sides.

2. In a food processor, combine the cashews, shredded coconut, coconut flour, dates, chia seeds, coffee, almond milk, vanilla, maple syrup, cocoa powder, cinnamon, and MCT oil. Process until completely granular. Pour the mixture into the prepared pan. Smooth out the top with a spatula.

3. Refrigerate for at least 2 hours or overnight, or until firm and set. Using the overhanging parchment as handles, remove the block from the pan and slice it into 2-inch squares.

4. Store in an airtight container in the refrigerator for up to 2 weeks.

+

DAIRY-FREE

GLUTEN-FREE

VEGAN

VEGETARIAN

BETTER DIGESTION

BETTER FOCUS

Private chef Mikaela Reuben spent time as a self-described "beach bum" in Maui before training in holistic nutrition, eventually going on the road with rock bands like Pearl Jam and Red Hot Chili Peppers. "I've traveled so much, I can pull on different herbs and culinary styles while keeping nutrition in mind," says the healthy cook. Mikaela shares this energizing mix to balance blood sugar and keep the snacking scaries at bay, sans chemicals and processed sugars; it's made savory with the briny taste of ume plum vinegar. "It's a great grab-and-go snack that I'm obsessed with," she writes (from the road, of course).

SPICED NUT MIX

Makes 3 cups

3 cups mixed raw almonds, cashews, and hazelnuts

2 tablespoons ume plum vinegar or red wine vinegar

½ teaspoon smoked paprika

1 teaspoon freshly ground black pepper

1 teaspoon onion powder

2 teaspoons black sesame seeds

¼ teaspoon dried oregano

1. Preheat the oven to 350°F. Line a baking sheet with parchment paper.

2. Spread the nuts over the prepared baking sheet, spacing them apart evenly. Toast for about 15 minutes, until fragrant and golden brown.

3. Quickly transfer the nuts to a large bowl (set the lined baking sheet aside). Immediately add the vinegar, paprika, pepper, onion powder, sesame seeds, and oregano to the bowl. Using a wooden spoon, stir to coat the nuts evenly.

4. Return the nuts to the baking sheet, spreading them out into an even layer, and let cool completely. Store in an airtight container at room temperature for up to 1 week.

+

DAIRY-FREE

GLUTEN-FREE

VEGAN

VEGETARIAN

BETTER ENERGY

BETTER FOCUS

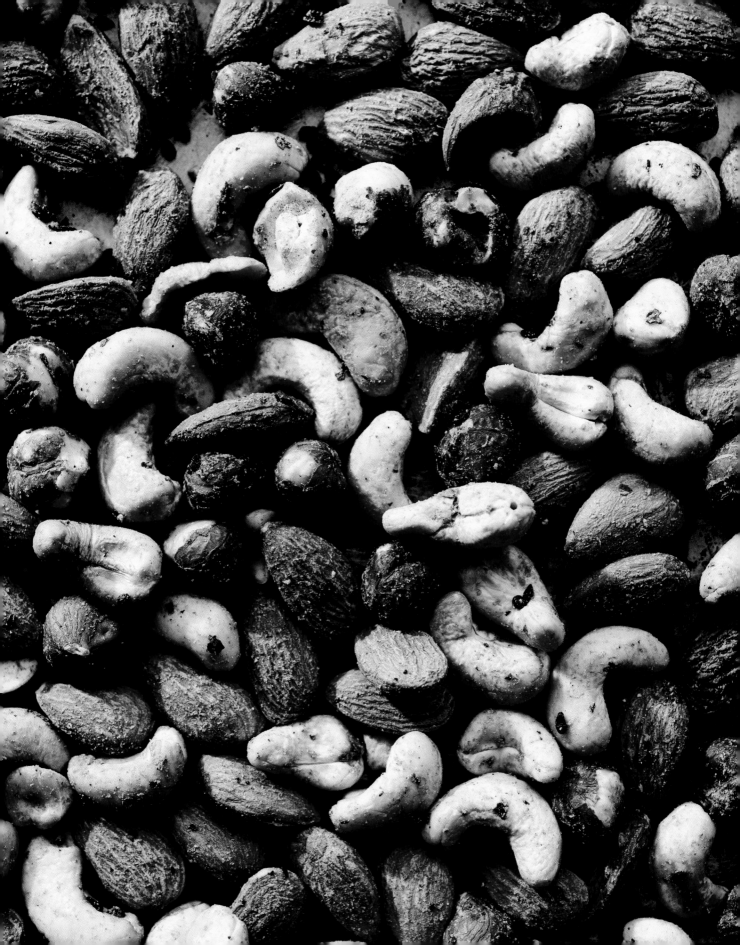

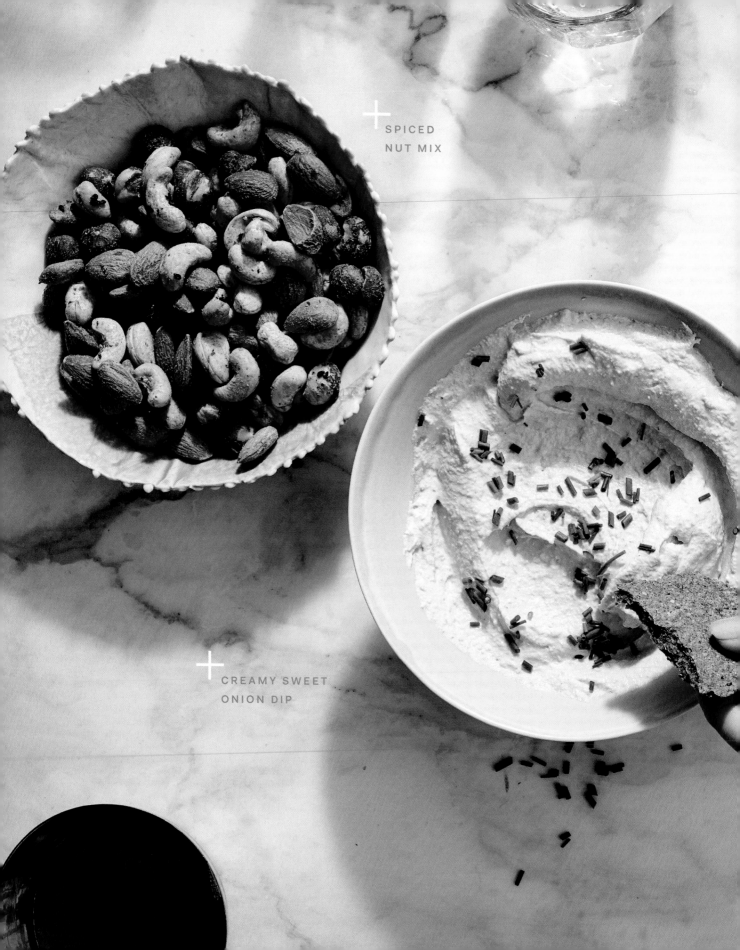

+ SPICED
NUT MIX

+ CREAMY SWEET
ONION DIP

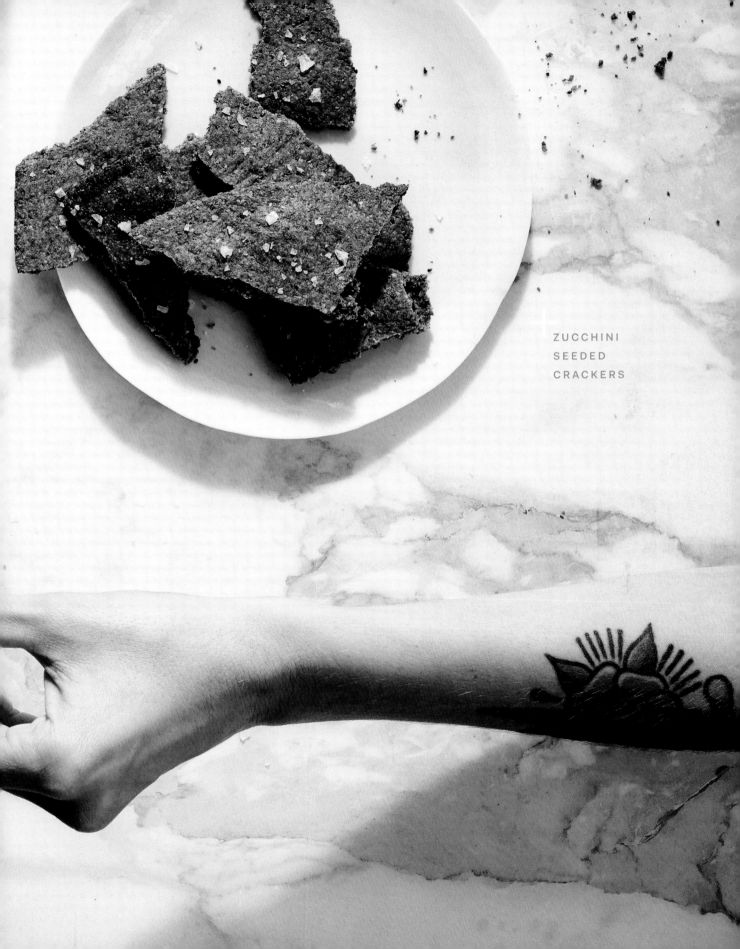

ZUCCHINI
SEEDED
CRACKERS

Nutritionist McKel Hill, MS, RDN, LDN, has made a career out of helping women to listen to their bodies and eat in a way that honors and supports their overall health and wellness. Well, sometimes, she realizes, your body cries out for that classic French onion dip that every parent served at every party (hey, childhood memories die hard). That's exactly what inspired this recipe—but in McKel's version, the delicious dip is packed with B vitamins and plant-based protein. Plus, she adds, "We can thank the cashews and olive oil for a nice boost of healthy fats." Save any leftovers of this dairy-free (yet totally creamy) spread and use it to dress up grain bowls and sandwiches.

CREAMY SWEET ONION DIP

Makes 1 cup

2 tablespoons olive oil, plus more as needed

2 medium to large red onions, thinly sliced (about 2 cups)

Sea salt and freshly ground black pepper

2 tablespoons nutritional yeast

Juice of ½ lemon

1 heaping cup raw cashews, soaked in water for at least 30 minutes or overnight, and drained

1½ teaspoons onion salt mix (or see Tip)

1 garlic clove, minced

Chopped fresh chives, to finish

DAIRY-FREE

GLUTEN-FREE

KETOGENIC

VEGAN

VEGETARIAN

BETTER ENERGY

BETTER FOCUS

1. Heat the oil in a large skillet over medium heat. When it shimmers, add the onions and season with sea salt and pepper. Cook, stirring, for about 5 minutes, until soft and translucent.

2. Reduce the heat to medium-low and cook, stirring occasionally, for 15 to 20 minutes more, until golden brown. If the onions begin to stick, add 1 to 2 tablespoons water and stir, scraping up the caramelized bits from the bottom of the pan. Cook until the onions are slightly purple but golden brown, about 15 minutes more. The onions will reduce significantly in volume and will smell and taste sweet.

3. Transfer the caramelized onions to a high-speed blender or food processor and add the nutritional yeast, lemon juice, cashews, onion salt mix, and garlic and blend until completely smooth. Transfer to a serving bowl and top with a drizzle of olive oil and the chopped chives.

4. Serve with Zucchini Seeded Crackers (opposite). Store leftover dip in an airtight container in the refrigerator for up to 1 week.

Tip: Make your own onion salt mix with 1 teaspoon each of granulated onion, granulated garlic, dried minced onion, sea salt, dried minced scallion, and dried chives.

Pediatric nutritionist and cookbook author Mandy Sacher's philosophy is simple: Train a child's taste buds early to establish good eating habits for life. "I'm a big advocate for taking family favorites and giving them a healthy overhaul to boost the nutritional content," says the founder of Wholesome Child, which aims to educate and empower families on their wellness journeys. These crackers are bursting with chia and flax seeds, making them a no-brainer alternative to store-bought crackers—and a staple in Mandy's lunchbox lineup for her kids (and herself).

ZUCCHINI SEEDED CRACKERS

Makes 12 crackers

⅓ cup raw pumpkin seeds

¼ cup flaxseed

¼ cup raw sunflower seeds

¼ cup white sesame seeds

¼ cup chia seeds

1 cup buckwheat flour or whole-grain flour of choice

½ cup finely grated zucchini

¼ cup extra-virgin olive oil

⅓ cup filtered water

1 teaspoon sea salt

1. Preheat the oven to 425°F.

2. In a food processor, combine the pumpkin, flax, sunflower, sesame, and chia seeds and pulse until smooth. Add the buckwheat flour, zucchini, olive oil, and filtered water and process until smooth but just combined. The dough should still be thick but easy to spread.

3. Turn out the dough onto a sheet of parchment paper and set another sheet on top. Roll the dough out to about ¼ inch thick. Remove the top sheet of parchment and transfer the dough on the bottom sheet of parchment to a baking sheet.

4. Sprinkle the sea salt on the dough. Bake for about 20 minutes, or until golden and crisp. Remove the baking sheet from the oven and set it on a wire rack. Let the crackers cool completely.

5. Break into pieces and serve immediately, or store in an airtight container at room temperature for up to 1 week or in the freezer for up to 4 months.

6. Serve with Creamy Sweet Onion Dip (opposite) or Turmeric-Tahini Yogurt Dip (page 220).

DAIRY-FREE

GLUTEN-FREE

KETOGENIC

LOW-FODMAP

LOW-INFLAMMATION

PALEO

VEGAN

VEGETARIAN

BETTER DIGESTION

BETTER ENERGY

BETTER SKIN

"I love a good hummus as much as the next person, but I was getting a bit tired of it," says Melissa Hemsley, one half of Hemsley + Hemsley, the London healthy food scene stars who started with a home delivery service and now have a café, cookbooks, and a TV show. This dip, which Melissa calls "the new hummus," doesn't require whipping out (or, more important, cleaning) a blender or food processor. Plus, there's no chopping of crudités, which means even less effort standing between you and a supercharged snack. Use coconut yogurt to keep things anti-inflammatory.

TURMERIC-TAHINI YOGURT DIP WITH ENDIVE

Makes 1 cup

2 heads endive, leaves separated

1 cup full-fat yogurt or vegan coconut yogurt

2 tablespoons light tahini

1 large garlic clove, minced

Juice of ½ lemon

½ teaspoon ground turmeric

Sea salt and freshly ground black pepper

Extra-virgin olive oil, for serving

Fresh parsley, for serving (optional)

1. Arrange the endive leaves on a platter.

2. In a medium bowl, whisk together the yogurt, tahini, garlic, lemon juice, and turmeric until smooth. Taste and season with salt and pepper as desired.

3. Transfer the dip to a serving bowl and top with a drizzle of olive oil and some parsley, if desired. Finish with a sprinkle each of salt and freshly cracked pepper, and serve alongside the endive leaves.

DAIRY-FREE

GLUTEN-FREE

LOW-INFLAMMATION

VEGAN

VEGETARIAN

BETTER MOOD

BETTER SKIN

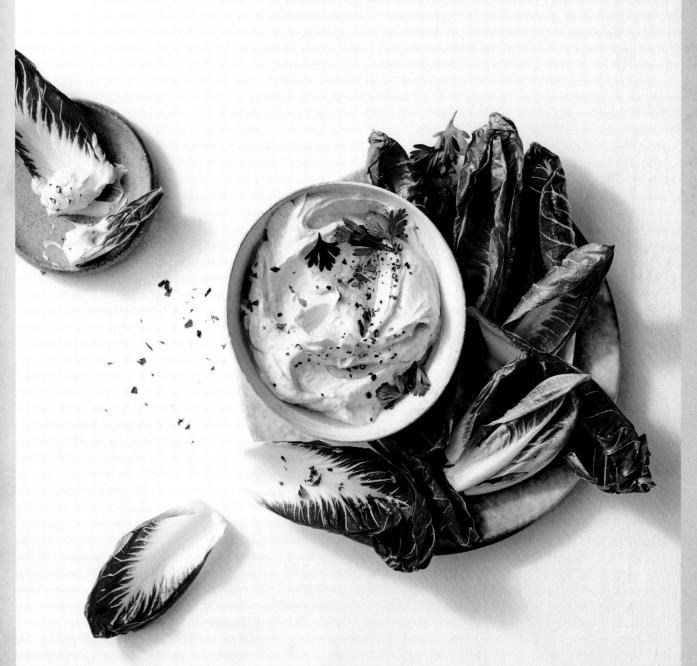

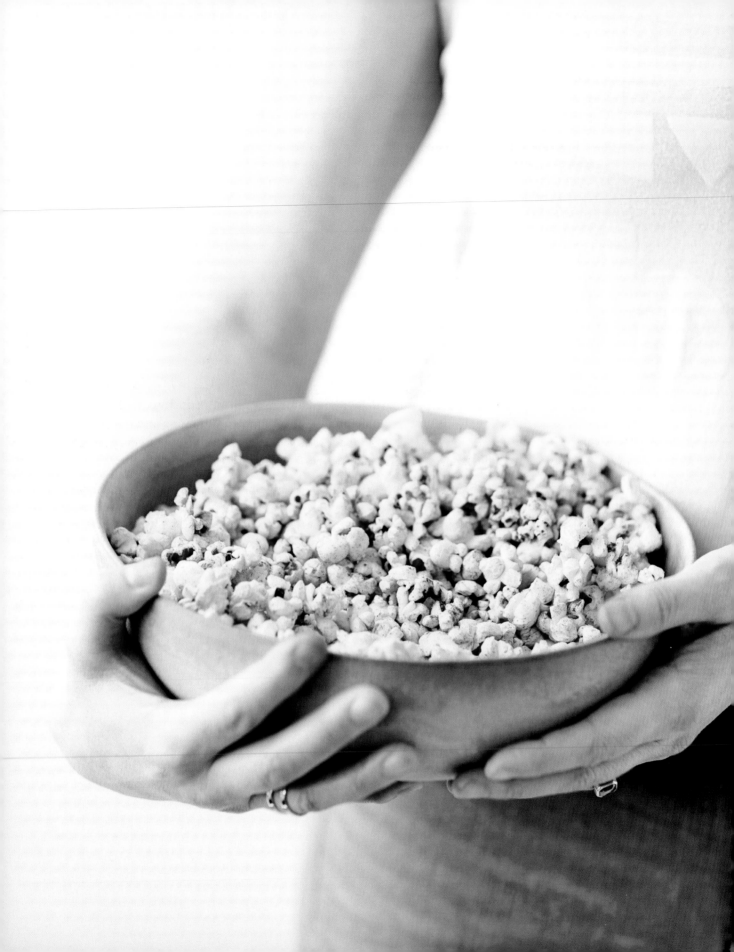

"If I can't pronounce everything on the ingredients label, it goes back on the shelf," says Well+Good food editor Emily Laurence. Take a cue from this former queen of processed foods (who became a home-cook enthusiast after converting to health journalism) and DIY your snacks with a touch of sweet-meets-spicy. "Seriously, when it comes to party prep, this one takes the gold," Emily says. Just keep it away from your white T-shirt.

COCONUT-TURMERIC POPCORN

Makes about 12 cups

¼ cup coconut oil

⅔ cup non-GMO popcorn kernels

1 teaspoon ground turmeric

1 teaspoon ground cinnamon

Sea salt to taste

1. Melt the coconut oil in a large pot over high heat. Add the popcorn kernels. Cover and wait for the kernels to begin to pop, then cook, shaking the pot vigorously to avoid burning, until the popcorn fills the pot and the time between pops slows to 2 to 3 seconds. Remove the pot from the heat and transfer the popcorn to a large bowl.

2. Sprinkle with the turmeric and cinnamon, season with salt, and enjoy.

DAIRY-FREE

GLUTEN-FREE

LOW-FODMAP

LOW-INFLAMMATION

VEGAN

VEGETARIAN

BETTER SKIN

COCKTAILS, COFFEES + TURBO-CHARGED TONICS

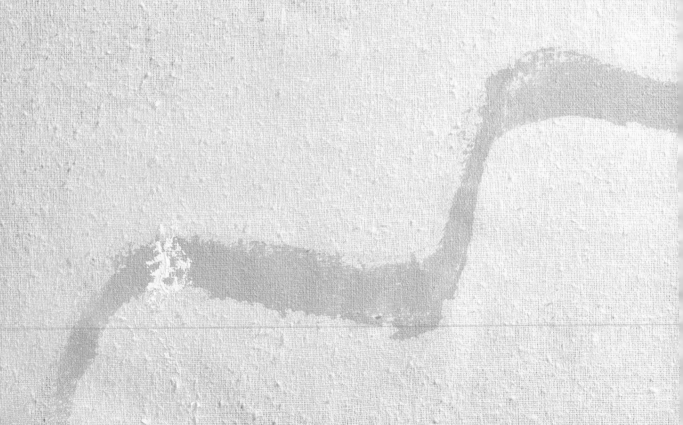

"A friend coming out of surgery asked me to make her some foods and juices for fast healing," says Lily Diamond. "This was the first one I gave her, for drinking pre- and post-op." The *Kale & Caramel* author says it's her favorite way to give the body a boost, with "the anti-inflammatory powers of fresh turmeric root and invigorating cayenne." Get ready to elevate your vitamin A and C intake for a sweet (and spicy) immunity-supporting sip. Add extra ice cubes at the end to turn this juice into more of a frozen slushy.

ORANGE ZINGER JUICE

Serves 2

1 (1-inch) piece fresh turmeric, peeled

1 (1-inch) piece fresh ginger, peeled (see Tip)

4 medium oranges, peeled and seeded

¼ to ½ lime, peeled and seeded

4 to 8 ice cubes (optional)

1. In a high-speed blender, combine the turmeric, ginger, oranges, lime, and ice cubes (if using). Blend until completely smooth.

2. Pour into two glasses and enjoy immediately.

Tip: Peel roots like ginger and turmeric easily using the edge of a spoon. Simply hold the knob in one hand and a spoon in the other, and drag the spoon's tip across the knob, applying pressure to scrape away the skin.

DAIRY-FREE

GLUTEN-FREE

LOW-INFLAMMATION

VEGAN

VEGETARIAN

BETTER DIGESTION

BETTER SKIN

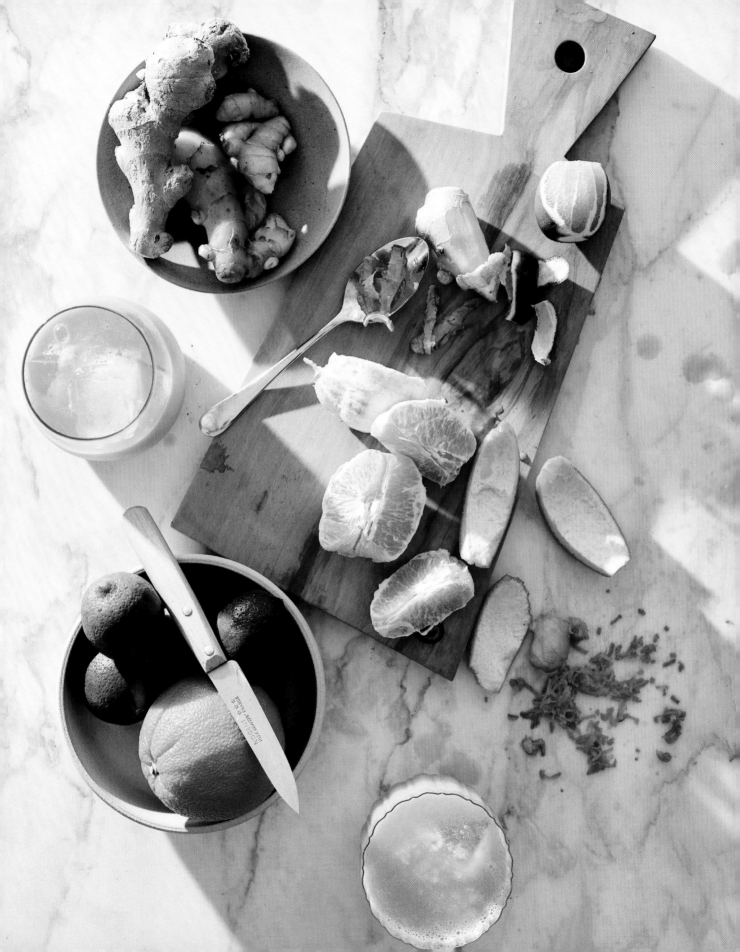

Wellness practitioner and herbalist Rachelle Robinett is passionate about the healing power of plants. She studied with specialists across the Americas before founding Supernatural, a New York City wellness café where she also practices herbalism. She uses this heartwarming brew to conjure affection among others, or for herself, and keeps a small selection of the herbs clearly visible in her daily life "as a reminder of love." Ask for damiana and skullcap at herbal shops, order them online, or skip the specialty ingredients altogether for an equally enjoyable potion. Debating the brandy? The alcohol and honey act as preservatives, allowing the brew to age gracefully: It keeps for 6 months.

LOVE POTION ELIXIR

Makes 5 cups

2 tablespoons ground cinnamon, or 2 cinnamon sticks

1 tablespoon pure vanilla extract

Zest of 1 orange, peeled with a vegetable peeler

4 cups filtered water

2 tablespoons cacao nibs

2 tablespoons food-grade hibiscus flowers

2 tablespoons food-grade rose hips

2 tablespoons damiana (optional)

2 tablespoons dried skullcap (optional)

2 cups raw honey

2 cups brandy (optional)

1. In a small saucepan, combine the cinnamon, vanilla, orange zest, filtered water, cacao nibs, hibiscus flowers, rose hips, damiana, and skullcap. Cover and bring to a simmer over low heat. Simmer for at least 1 hour, until fragrant. (For a stronger potion, simmer, uncovered, until the liquid has reduced by half.)

2. Strain the liquid through cheesecloth or a fine-mesh sieve into a glass jar; discard the solids. Let cool slightly (it should be warm, not hot), then add the honey and stir until it has dissolved. Add the brandy (if using) and stir to combine.

3. Cover and store in the refrigerator for up to 6 months. When ready to serve, pour ½ cup of the elixir into a small saucepan, reheat, and serve in a small glass, or skip the reheating and serve chilled over ice.

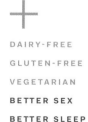

DAIRY-FREE

GLUTEN-FREE

VEGETARIAN

BETTER SEX

BETTER SLEEP

LAUREN SINGER

Zero-waste guru Lauren Singer can fit all the trash she's produced over the past four years into *one* 16-ounce mason jar—but she also keeps a few extra jars around to make this recipe, her signature cocktail. "This is my party go-to—it's foolproof, takes only twenty-four hours, and makes a damn good Dark and Stormy," says the creator of the *Trash Is for Tossers* blog and founder of Brooklyn's Package Free Shop. Experiment with subbing in the juice from an orange (bought from a farmer's market, sans packaging, of course) for the lemon juice, to switch up the flavor.

GINGER BEER

Makes 8 cups

2 cups coarsely chopped peeled fresh ginger (see Tip, page 226)

2 cups sugar

Juice of 2 medium lemons (about ¼ cup)

1 tablespoon active dry yeast

1. Bring 8 cups water to boil in a large pot over high heat.

2. In a large glass container, such as a 1-gallon mason jar, combine the ginger, sugar, and the boiling water and stir well to dissolve the sugar. Stir in the lemon juice. Let the mixture cool slightly, about 5 minutes. Add the yeast and stir to dissolve.

3. Cover with cheesecloth or a clean kitchen towel and let sit on the counter for 24 hours to brew. Strain the mixture and transfer to the refrigerator to chill until ready to drink, up to 1 week.

> **Tip:** Pair with a lime for a mocktail, or mix with rum, simple syrup, and lime juice for Lauren's favorite Dark and Stormy—but either way, be sure to skip the plastic straw.

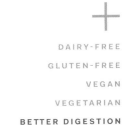

DAIRY-FREE

GLUTEN-FREE

VEGAN

VEGETARIAN

BETTER DIGESTION

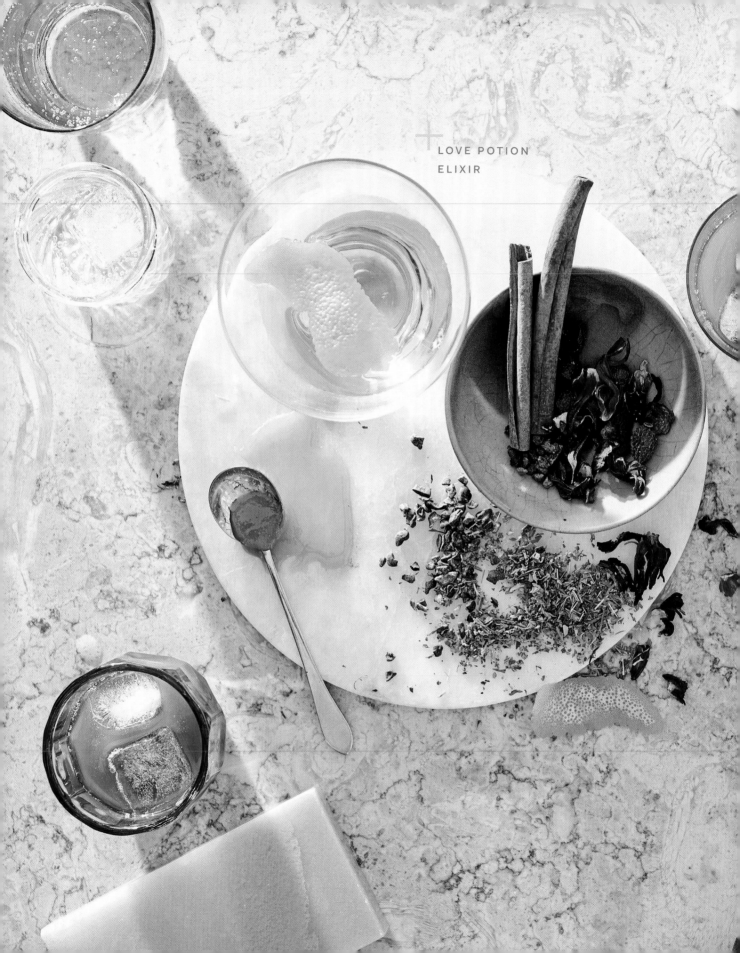

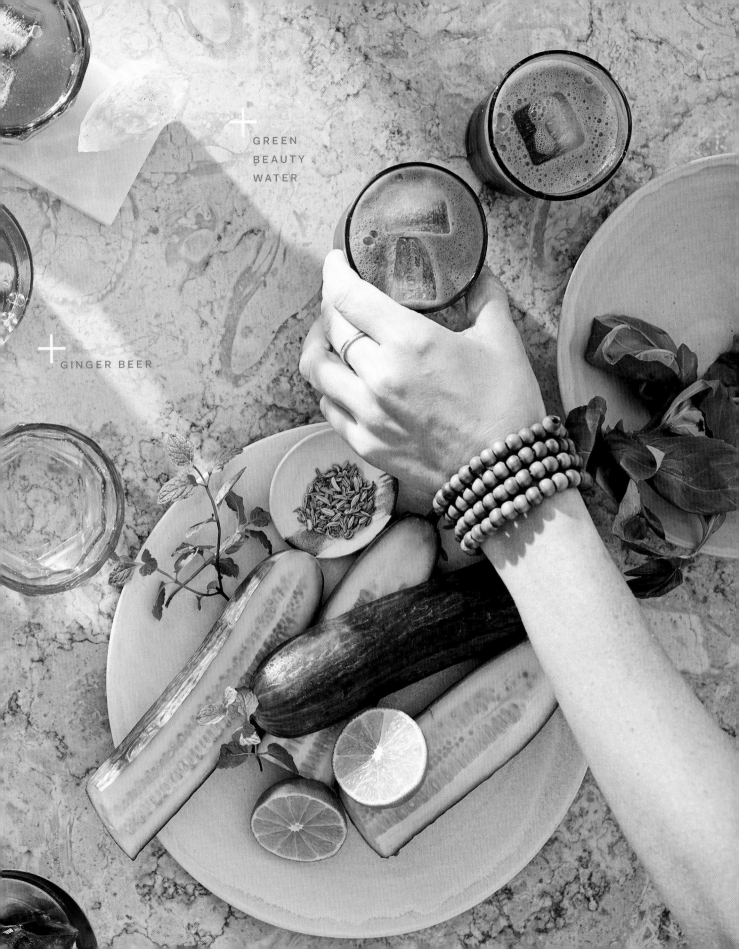

GREEN
BEAUTY
WATER

GINGER BEER

Ayurvedic doctor and holistic skincare expert Pratima Raichur frequently makes a big batch of this refreshing tonic to sip all day long. "It's a convenient way to consume more water throughout the day, while at the same time helping to boost immunity, stimulate metabolism, and promote collagen production," says the founder of New York City's Pratima Spa and its line of skincare products. It's her go-to suggestion for clients looking for clear skin, deep hydration, and balanced digestion. Refrigerate all the ingredients for at least two hours prior to making the drink so the flavors have a chance to shine.

GREEN BEAUTY WATER

Serves 4

4 cups filtered water

1 cucumber, peeled and seeded

½ teaspoon fennel seeds

8 large or 12 small fresh basil leaves

20 fresh mint leaves

Juice of 1 lime or lemon

1. In a high-speed blender, combine the filtered water, cucumber, fennel seeds, basil, mint, and lime juice. Blend for 1 minute, just until smooth. Taste—the liquid should be lightly flavored, with no one ingredient standing out; adjust the flavors as needed and blend again until smooth.

2. Strain the liquid through cheesecloth or a fine-mesh sieve into a large mason jar with a lid; discard the solids.

3. Pour into glasses and serve cold, or cover the jar and store in the refrigerator for up to 3 days.

DAIRY-FREE

GLUTEN-FREE

KETOGENIC

LOW-FODMAP

LOW-INFLAMMATION

PALEO

VEGAN

VEGETARIAN

BETTER FOCUS

BETTER SKIN

"I like to incorporate beneficial botanicals into every aspect of my life—even my cocktails," says Laura Silverman, the founding naturalist of the Outside Institute, which connects people to the healing and transformative powers of the natural world. Laura's mission to forage and source the most pristine local ingredients for her inventive, delicious, and lovingly prepared offerings is reflected in the earthiness of this cocktail. The Heartbeet is rich in antioxidants from beet juice and heart-healthy from the hibiscus, while the chili bitters help aid digestion. And the mezcal? "That's good for the soul," she says.

HEARTBEET COCKTAIL

Serves 1

2 ounces mezcal

1 ounce brewed and chilled hibiscus tea

½ to 1 ounce agave nectar

1 ounce red beet juice

Dash of chili bitters (optional)

Red beet slice, for garnish

1. Fill a cocktail shaker with ice. Add the mezcal, hibiscus tea, agave, beet juice, and bitters (if using). Shake until well chilled.

2. Pour into a rocks glass. Garnish with the beet slice and enjoy.

+

DAIRY-FREE

GLUTEN-FREE

VEGAN

VEGETARIAN

BETTER DIGESTION

Natural beauty expert, herbalist, and celeb makeup artist Jessa Blades drinks this immune-boosting tonic to stay healthy, thanks to ingredients like ginger, honey, and elderberry, which has long been used as a holistic remedy to help treat colds and flu. "This is a recipe that everyone should have up their sleeves," she says. In addition to the potent ingredients, the deep-purple elderberry syrup is *gorgeous*—leave it to a beauty pro to make fighting the common cold look glamorous. And one extra perk: You can store the leftover syrup in your fridge, to dress up anything bubbly.

ELDERBERRY-ROSEMARY SPRITZER

Makes 1 drink

1 to 2 tablespoons Elderberry Syrup (recipe follows)

Seltzer

1 rosemary sprig, for garnish

1 lemon round, for garnish

1. Fill a highball glass with ice. Add the syrup, then top with seltzer, taking care not to disturb the syrup at the bottom. Slap the rosemary sprig between your hands to activate its essential oils, then add it to the glass.

2. Garnish with a lemon round on the side of the glass (or let it float on top of the drink). Enjoy.

DAIRY-FREE

GLUTEN-FREE

LOW-INFLAMMATION

VEGETARIAN

BETTER ENERGY

BETTER FOCUS

ELDERBERRY SYRUP

Makes 5 to 6 cups

1 cup dried elderberries, or 2 cups fresh

2 cinnamon sticks

1 teaspoon whole cloves

1 teaspoon ground ginger, or 2 tablespoons grated fresh ginger

1 tablespoon dried orange peel, or ¼ cup fresh orange zest

1 tablespoon food-grade dried rose hips

½ teaspoon food-grade dried hibiscus

10 black cardamom pods

2 cups honey

1. In a large saucepan, combine the elderberries, cinnamon sticks, cloves, ginger, orange peel, rose hips, hibiscus, cardamom, and 5 cups water. Bring to a boil over medium-high heat, then reduce the heat to low and simmer for 25 minutes, until the mixture reaches a syrup-like consistency.

2. Strain the liquid through cheesecloth or a fine-mesh sieve into a large jar with a lid, pressing all of the liquid out of the berries with the back of a wooden spoon; discard the solids. Let cool for 5 minutes, then add the honey and stir until it has dissolved.

3. Cover and refrigerate for at least 2 hours or overnight, until cool. Store in the refrigerator for up to 3 months.

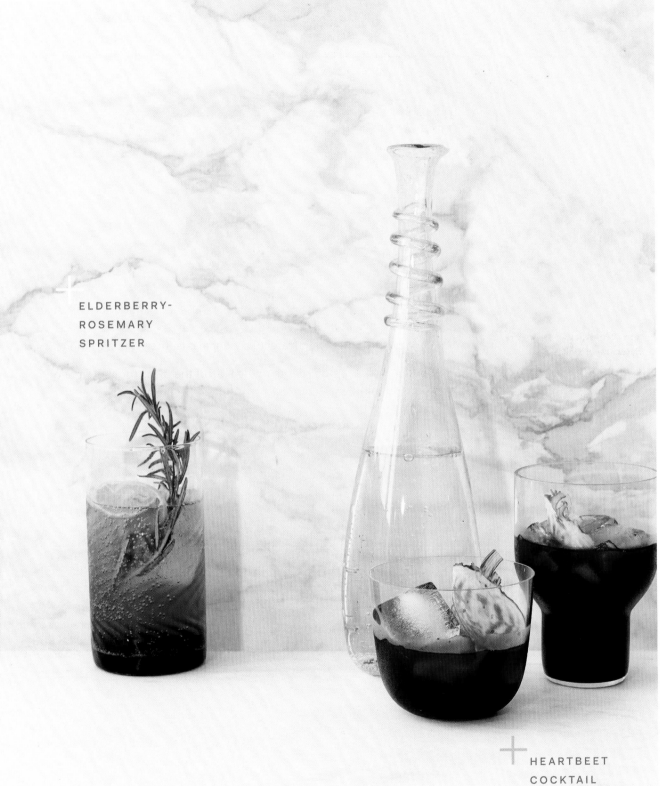

ELDERBERRY-
ROSEMARY
SPRITZER

HEARTBEET
COCKTAIL

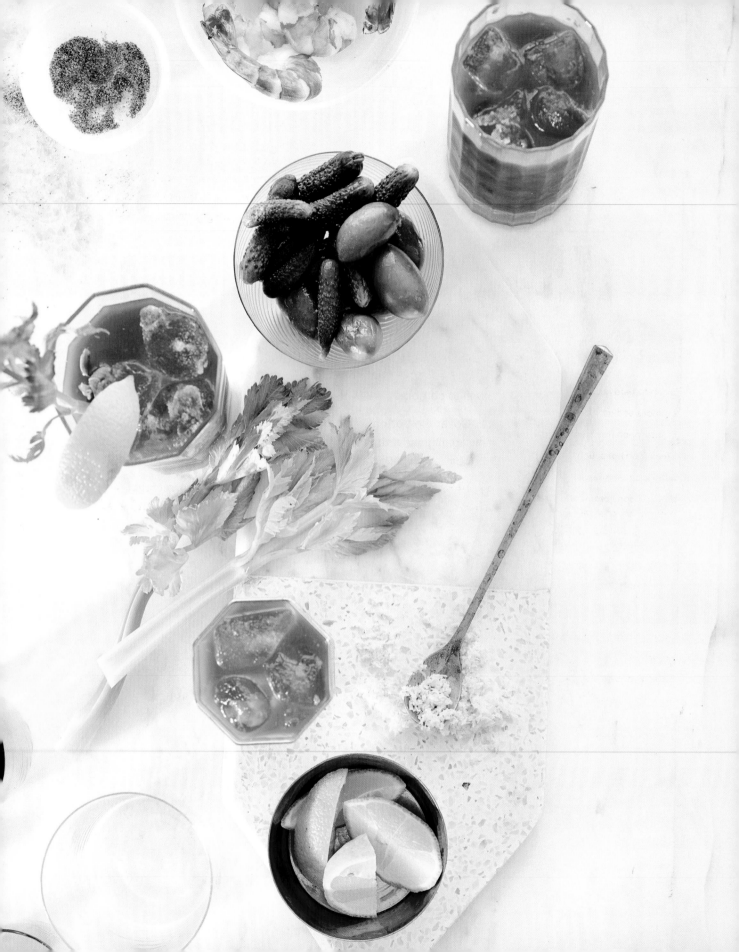

You may be surprised to learn that Bloody Marys are a part of fitness mogul Anna Kaiser's healthy lifestyle. As the founder of the ever-expanding mega dance cardio methods AKT and AKT on Demand, Anna (who trains Shakira and Kelly Ripa) sees this as part of her "80 percent on-track" ethos. "Cutting anything completely out of your diet is a recipe for disaster—that's all you end up wanting," she says of allowing for a little flexibility 20 percent of the time. Plus, vodka is considered a low-sugar alcohol. Anna loves celery salt, fresh shrimp, and lots of hot sauce added to her Bloody—feel free to get creative with the garnishes.

DIY BLOODY MARY BAR

Serves 1

¾ cup tomato juice

2 ounces vodka

1 tablespoon fresh lemon juice

1 teaspoon hot sauce

½ teaspoon kosher salt

1½ teaspoons prepared horseradish, or to taste

¼ teaspoon Worcestershire sauce

Celery salt

Ice cubes, for serving

GARNISHES

Lemon wedge

3 olives

2 cornichons

2 shrimp, cooked, peeled, and deveined

1 small celery stalk

1. In a cocktail shaker, combine the tomato juice, vodka, lemon juice, hot sauce, kosher salt, horseradish, and Worcestershire sauce. Shake well to combine.

2. Cover the bottom of a small dish with celery salt. Rub the rim of a highball glass with 1 lemon wedge, then dip the rim in the celery salt to coat. Add ice to the glass and pour the Bloody Mary over to top.

3. Use a toothpick to spear the lemon wedge, olives, cornichons, and shrimp and set the skewer on the rim of the glass or in the drink. Add the celery stick. Cheers to yourself and enjoy.

DAIRY-FREE

GLUTEN-FREE

As a wellness writer, recipe developer, and personal trainer, Tatiana Boncompagni spends most of her time in full-on health-geek mode—but she can also make a mean cocktail. This reimagined piña colada takes the classic drink into nondairy territory. Plus, "It's criminally delicious," Tatiana promises. You can easily make the tropical recipe more distinctively nutty by using almond milk creamer instead of the coconut milk version.

COCONUT RUM COLADA

Serves 2

1 cup salted roasted almonds

½ cup coconut milk creamer

½ cup pure maple syrup

4 ounces spiced rum

3 cups ice

2 star anise pods, for garnish

Ground cinnamon, for garnish

1. In a high-speed blender, combine the almonds, coconut milk creamer, maple syrup, rum, and 1 cup of the ice. Blend for 30 seconds, or until smooth. Add the remaining 2 cups ice and blend for 5 seconds more, until frothy.

2. Divide the drink between two highball glasses and garnish each with a star anise pod and a sprinkle of cinnamon. Serve immediately.

Tip: To prep this ahead of time, pour the drink into ice cube trays and freeze. When ready to serve, blend quickly for 2 to 5 seconds, until frosty.

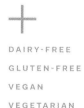

DAIRY-FREE

GLUTEN-FREE

VEGAN

VEGETARIAN

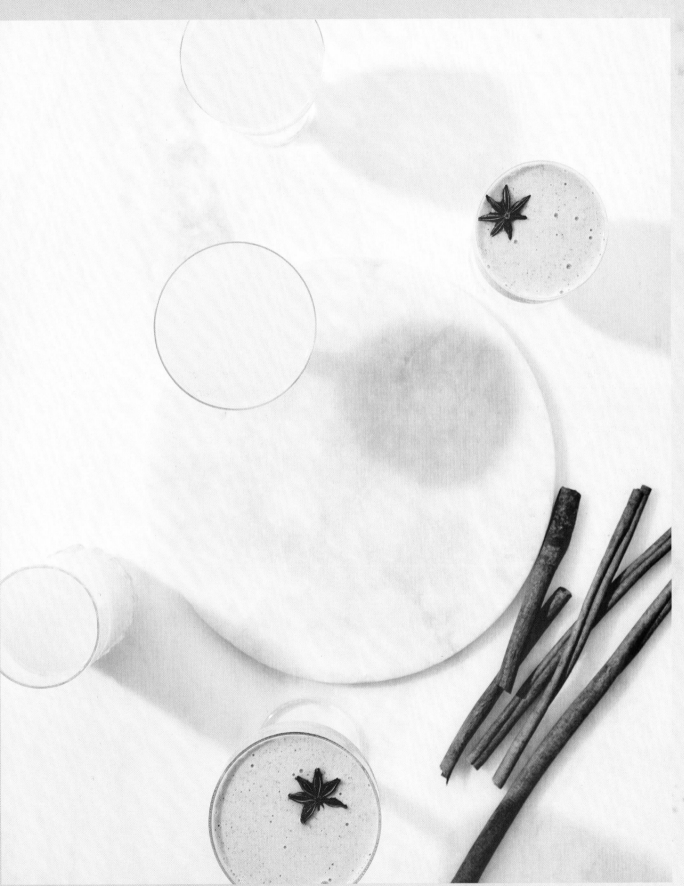

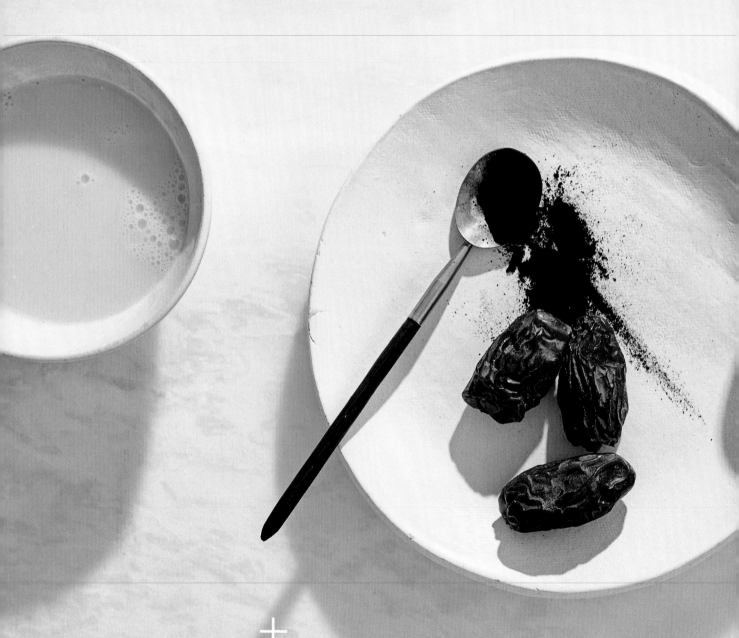

ACTIVATED
CHARCOAL LATTE

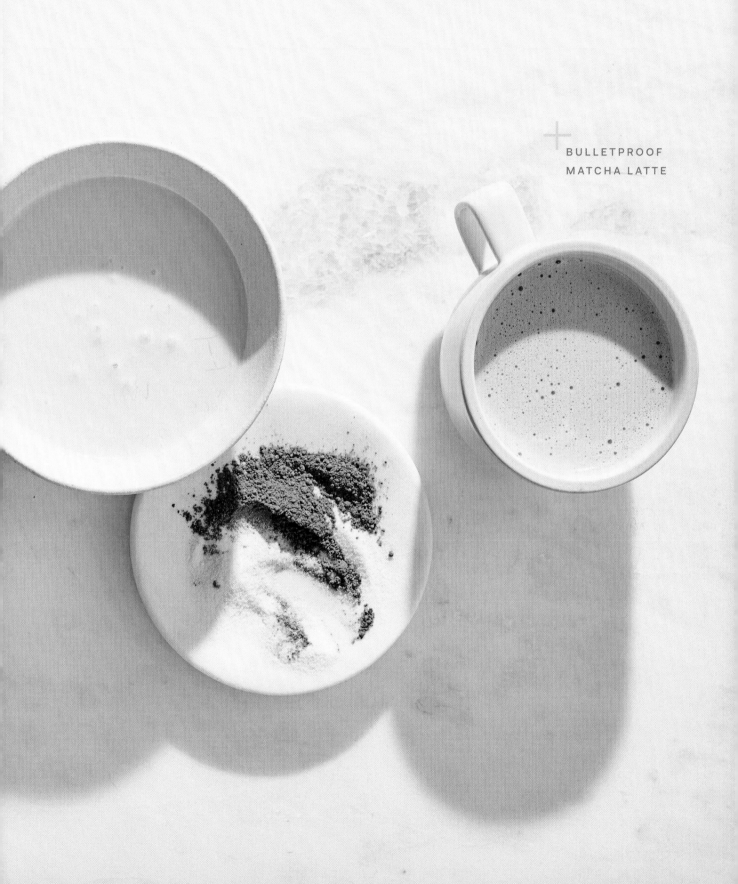

Ready for your new mantra? "Eat like you love yourself," says Nikisha Brunson, cofounder of the lifestyle blog *Urban Bush Babes*. The Toronto-born, Brooklyn-raised holistic maven and self-described "ex–teen mom" became obsessed with all-natural beauty and wellness over a decade ago, leading her to launch Folie Apothecary, a small-batch natural skincare and haircare line. With this warming cuppa, the detoxing activated charcoal (available at health food stores and online) blends perfectly into date-sweetened nut milk. Sip this latte with the awareness that charcoal pulls out nutrients and helpful medications as well as the stuff you don't want.

ACTIVATED CHARCOAL LATTE

Serves 1

1½ cups unsweetened almond milk or other nondairy milk

1 or 2 pitted dates, such as Medjool or Deglet Noor

½ teaspoon activated charcoal

1 teaspoon pure vanilla extract

1. In a small saucepan, combine the almond milk and dates. Heat over medium-high heat until steaming, about 4 minutes.

2. Carefully transfer the warm milk to a high-speed blender. Add the charcoal and vanilla and blend until creamy and frothy. Pour into a mug and serve hot.

DAIRY-FREE

GLUTEN-FREE

LOW-INFLAMMATION

VEGAN

VEGETARIAN

BETTER DIGESTION

Yes, it's true: The man behind Bulletproof Coffee (aka the reason everyone suddenly started putting grass-fed butter and MCT oil in their morning mug) sometimes switches up his sips. When Bulletproof 360 founder and CEO Dave Asprey doesn't want a full-on java jolt, he opts for this matcha latte, which provides a generous dose of antioxidants and healthy fats—and it's the perfect canvas for sneaking in some collagen protein. "I tend to rely on it at home as a late-afternoon pick-me-up before hiking with my family or working into the night," Dave says. Heads up: We think this recipe is totally sweet enough without the sugar substitute, but give your taste buds what they want.

BULLETPROOF MATCHA LATTE

Serves 1

1 cup coconut milk

½ cup boiling filtered water

1 teaspoon matcha green tea powder

1 teaspoon vanilla powder

2 tablespoons collagen powder (optional)

Stevia or hardwood xylitol (optional)

1. In a small saucepan, bring the coconut milk to a boil over medium-high heat, then immediately remove the pan from the heat. Pour the coconut milk into a blender.

2. In a measuring cup, whisk together the boiling water and the matcha to dissolve the powder, then pour the mixture into the blender with the coconut milk.

3. Add the vanilla powder and blend until the mixture has a creamy consistency and a layer of foam on top. Add the collagen powder (if using) and blend until it is incorporated. Taste and sweeten with stevia as desired.

4. Pour into a mug and serve hot.

+

DAIRY-FREE

GLUTEN-FREE

KETOGENIC

LOW-INFLAMMATION

PALEO

BETTER ENERGY

BETTER FOCUS

EAT FOR BETTER SLEEP

The Thanksgiving turkey has long held the title of "Food Most Likely to Make You Fall Asleep." And it's kind of a shame, because that totally stuffed holiday dinner isn't exactly something you'd want to replicate on a nightly basis if you regularly have trouble getting your z's. Fortunately, there's scientific data behind other healthy functional foods—without the buffet-table baggage—that can help relax you and set the stage for a really good night's sleep.

> HEALTHY FUNCTIONAL FOODS CAN HELP RELAX YOU AND SET THE STAGE FOR A REALLY GOOD NIGHT'S SLEEP.

Some of these sleepytime foods, like chicken, eggs, fish, yogurt, and cheese, contain tryptophan, the same amino acid found in turkey that the body uses to produce serotonin (a relaxation neurochemical) and melatonin (a sleepiness hormone that comes out when the sun goes down). When eaten with a few carbs—note that I said "a few"—tryptophan can spark your serotonin and cross the blood-brain barrier to help work its sleep-inducing magic.

Lately, in the wellness world, minerals like magnesium have stolen the spotlight (er, the nightlight?) as sleep-enhancers, which is why add-to-water calming magnesium powders and rub-on-your-belly magnesium oils have been flying off natural food store shelves. This idea comes from initial promising evidence that magnesium reduces adrenaline levels, and helps relax the mind and body. Similarly, a few small studies have suggested that a lack of calcium in your diet can lead to nighttime awakenings.

Compared to powering down your devices hours before bed, which a lot of people admittedly find really, really challenging, eating for better sleep is relatively simple. Here are some of my top tips for how to do it. Keep things consistent, and you'll reap the benefits—day and night.

NO HEAVY MEALS OR ALCOHOL WITHIN THREE HOURS OF BEDTIME. Large, heavy, spicy meals can lead to reflux and stomach upset. The same goes for foods that are high in saturated fat and sugar or low in fiber. Wine with dinner always sounds like a great idea, and may make you sleepy initially, but alcohol also causes more nighttime awakenings and morning grogginess.

HAVE A *SMALL* SLEEP SNACK ONE HOUR BEFORE BED. Combine a tryptophan-containing protein with a complex carbohydrate, like Greek yogurt with nut butter and banana, or a few pieces of cheese and whole-grain or rice crackers.

EAT FOODS RICH IN MAGNESIUM AND CALCIUM TO HELP DIAL DOWN YOUR ADRENALINE. Nuts, seeds, yogurt, avocado, and fish all contain magnesium. Many of these foods also contain calcium, as do almond milk, dark leafy greens, broccoli, dairy products, oranges, chickpeas, sardines, and sustainable salmon.

FILL YOUR PLATE WITH FOODS THAT BOOST YOUR BRAIN'S MELATONIN PRODUCTION. Tart cherry juice, oats, barley, flaxseed, sunflower seeds, peanuts, bananas, grapes, cucumber, and broccoli are all great choices that research shows may help tossing and turning.

—SHELBY HARRIS, PSYD

MARIE KONDO

Ever since she was a child, Marie Kondo has loved sipping *amazake*, a fermented Japanese rice drink, found in shops adjacent to many Japanese shrines. "It helps me relax and warms me from the core when I'm tired," says the decluttering guru, whose 2014 book *The Life-Changing Magic of Tidying Up* made her a worldwide star. "Relaxing" is something she has to slot into her calendar these days—and Marie has learned how to make the drink at home, experimenting with various recipes before settling on this one. Her husband, Takumi, blends the *amazake* with milk and banana for a cold treat.

AMAZAKE

Makes 4 cups

½ cup cooked white rice

4 ounces rice koji (see Tip)

1. In a thermal pot or cooker, combine the cooked rice and 1½ cups water and mix well with a wooden spoon. Add the koji crumbles, which start the fermentation process, and stir to combine thoroughly.

2. Let the mixture sit for 8 to 12 hours in the 130 to 150°F range, stirring occasionally and maintaining the temperature at all times.

3. Increase the temperature to 167°F or higher to stop the fermentation and prevent the amazake from becoming sour. It will resemble a rice-flecked, super-runny porridge.

4. Pour the mixture into a mug and serve hot. Store the amazake in an airtight container in the refrigerator for up to 1 week.

Tip: Koji is a bacterial culture that's been added to barley or rice and is used to make fermented foods; it's the same principle as a sourdough-bread starter. Koji can be ordered online or found in Japanese grocery stores and typically comes dried.

DAIRY-FREE

GLUTEN-FREE

LOW-FODMAP

LOW-INFLAMMATION

VEGAN

VEGETARIAN

BETTER DIGESTION

BETTER SLEEP

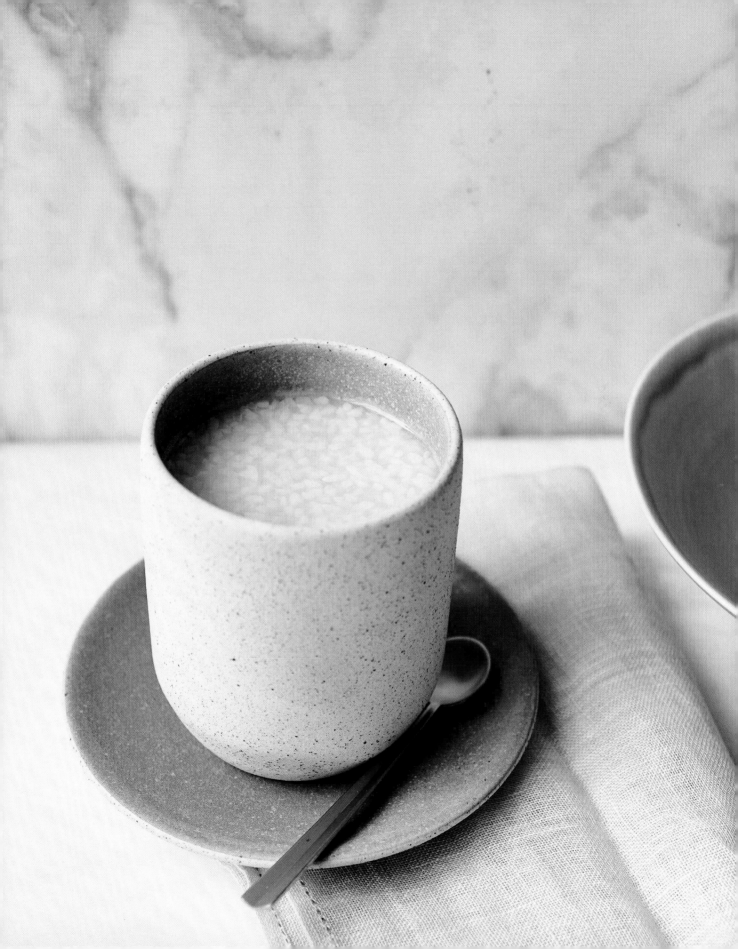

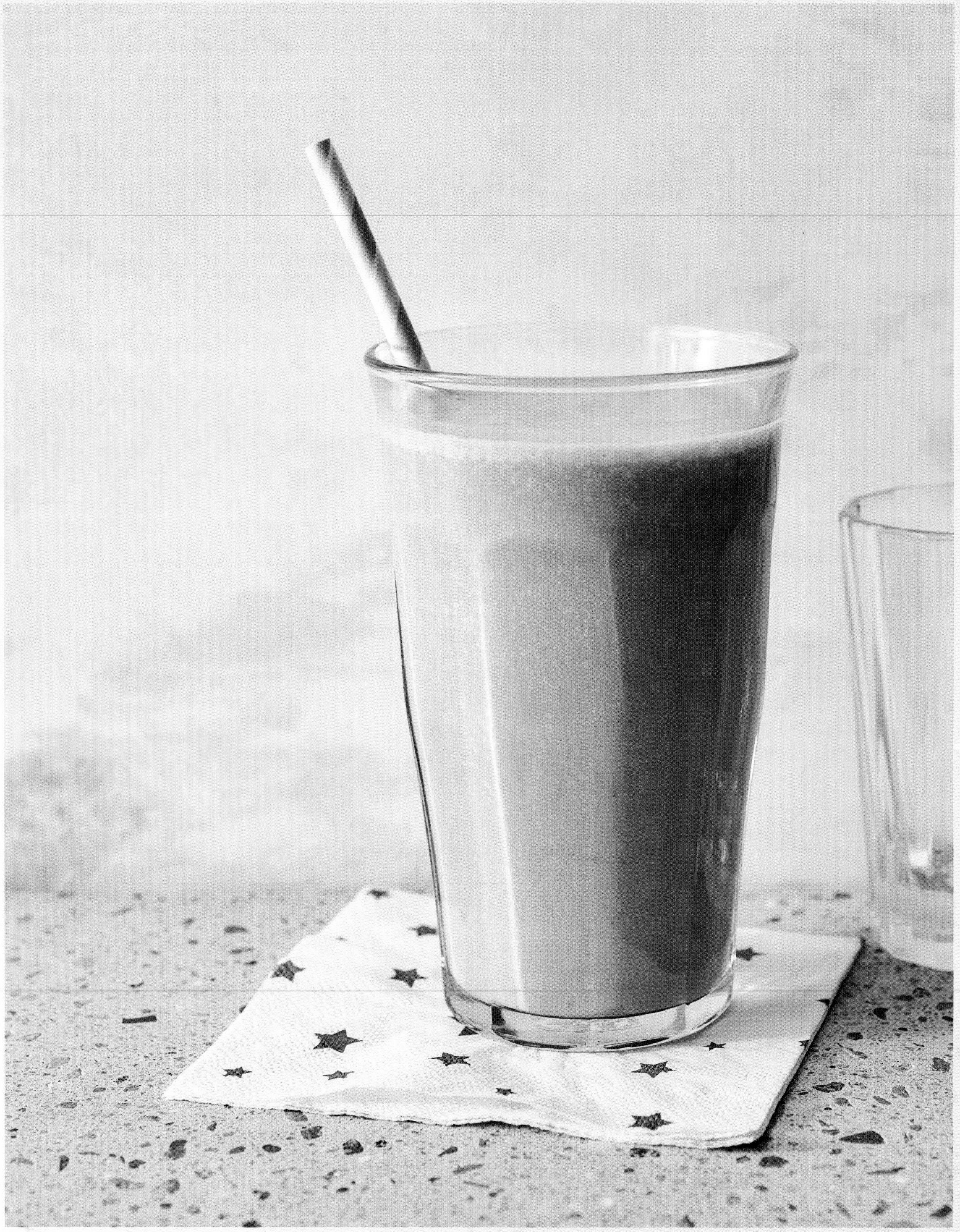

As a marathon runner who recently started to work on more strength training, Shelby Harris, PsyD, is all in on micellar casein protein powder, especially right before bed. "A milk-based protein, casein (also found in cottage cheese and Greek yogurt) is slow-digesting and works best when your muscles have a long time to rest, feeding them overnight and keeping you full as well," says Dr. Harris, who specializes in sleep issues. The almond milk and banana are rich in tryptophan (which helps your brain naturally produce melatonin) and magnesium (a deficiency in which can lead to poor sleep, too). Oats have slow-digesting carbs to help your brain produce relaxing serotonin, as well.

SWEET DREAMS SHAKE

Serves 1

1 cup unsweetened almond milk, chilled

¼ cup mashed ripe banana (about ½ banana)

2 tablespoons instant oats, softened in 2 tablespoons warm water for 2 minutes

2 to 3 tablespoons chocolate micellar casein protein powder (see Tip)

1. In a blender, combine the almond milk, banana, oats, and casein powder. Blend until smooth and creamy.

2. Pour into a tall glass and enjoy.

Tip: Use a casein powder that doesn't have any added sleep-inducing ingredients (e.g., melatonin). Stick to micellar casein, which can be found online or in health food or supplement stores.

VEGETARIAN

BETTER SKIN

BETTER SLEEP

"Good karma served daily" is the motto at Inday, New York City's fave fast-casual, Indian-inspired eatery. Its founder, Basu Ratnam, created this invigorating, feel-good drink for the restaurant based on an old family recipe. "We grew up drinking chai infused with warming herbs and spices—toasting and grinding them into a special blend (called a *masala*)," says the former Fortune 500 finance consultant. This DIY-chai is everything you need in the morning or for a midafternoon boost, especially with the healthy twist of fatty-acid-friendly coconut milk.

WAKE-UP MASALA CHAI

Serves 1

2¼ teaspoons plus
⅛ teaspoon honey

⅜ teaspoon coriander seeds

⅜ teaspoon green cardamom pods

³⁄₁₆ teaspoon fennel seeds

⅛ teaspoon freshly grated or ground cinnamon

1½ teaspoons grated fresh ginger

1 teaspoon loose Assam tea leaves

1¼ teaspoons coconut milk

1. Bring a kettle of water to a boil over high heat.

2. In a medium bowl, stir together 2¼ teaspoons of the honey, the coriander seeds, cardamom pods, fennel seeds, cinnamon, and ginger. Add ½ cup of the boiling water from the kettle and whisk to combine. Let steep for 2 minutes; return the kettle to a boil.

3. Add another ½ cup of the boiling water and the tea leaves and whisk to combine. Let steep for 2 minutes more. Pour the remaining boiling water into a mug to warm it.

4. Whisk the coconut milk into the bowl with the tea.

5. Discard the water from the mug. Strain the chai through a tea or cocktail strainer into the warmed mug. Enjoy.

DAIRY-FREE

GLUTEN-FREE

LOW-INFLAMMATION

VEGETARIAN

BETTER DIGESTION

BETTER FOCUS

BETTER SKIN

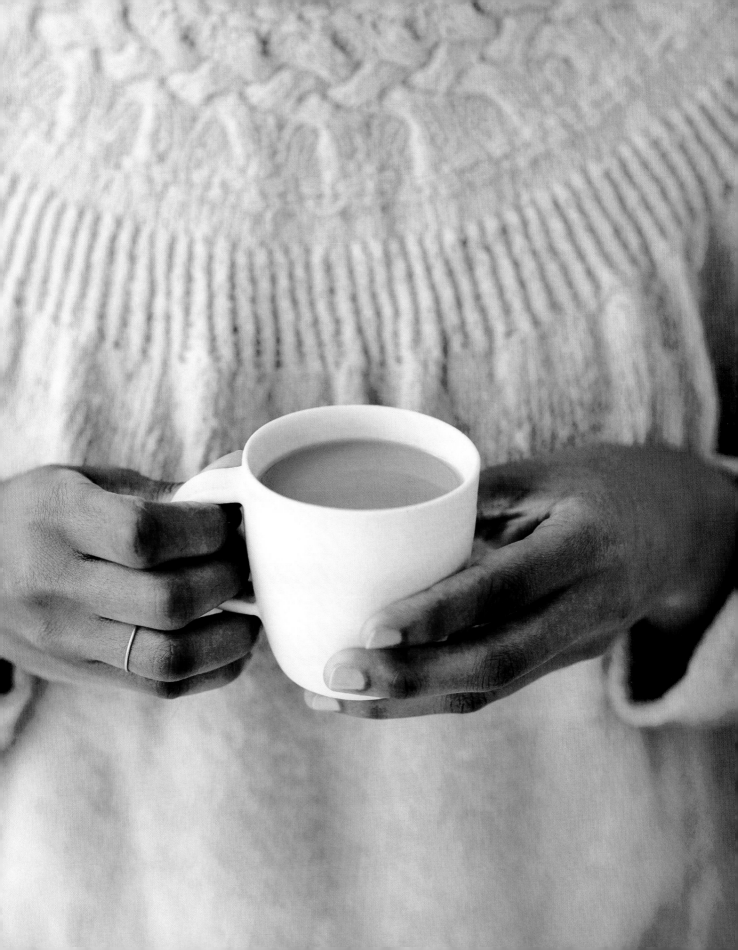

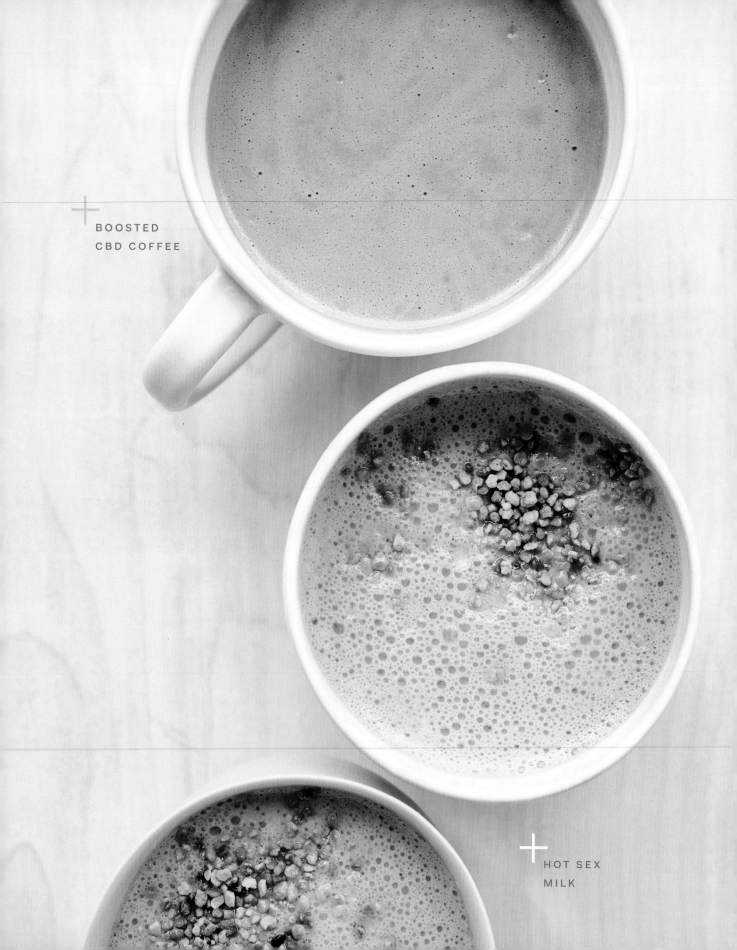

BOOSTED
CBD COFFEE

HOT SEX
MILK

It wasn't until she'd graduated from Harvard Business School and moved to Los Angeles to help elevate the cannabis industry that Jessica Assaf learned the health benefits of boosted coffee. Fats and caffeine bind together for focus and satiety, sure, but then "value-added ingredients" take it up another notch, with maca for energy, collagen for nail and hair health, and a splash of CBD oil for mental calm and clarity, explains Jessica, the founder of Cannabis Feminist, a female-led cannabis community, and cofounder of a hemp-based wellness company. She finds deep pleasure in the slow act of making this drink as a daily morning ritual.

BOOSTED CBD COFFEE

Serves 1

¾ cup hot brewed coffee

2 tablespoons coconut oil, ghee, or grass-fed butter (or a combination)

1 tablespoon grass-fed or fish-based collagen powder

1 teaspoon maca powder

1 teaspoon raw cacao powder

1 drop unflavored CBD oil (about 5 mg)

1 teaspoon pure maple syrup, honey, coconut sugar, or date sugar (optional)

1. In a blender, combine the coffee, coconut oil, collagen powder, maca, cacao, CBD oil, and maple syrup (if using). Blend on low for about 30 seconds, until the ingredients bind to the coffee and the coffee appears lighter in color, then increase the speed to high and blend for a few seconds more, until the mixture froths.

2. Pour the boosted coffee into a mug and enjoy hot, or serve over ice.

+

GLUTEN-FREE

KETOGENIC

LOW-FODMAP

LOW-INFLAMMATION

PALEO

BETTER FOCUS

BETTER MOOD

Before starting Moon Juice, a juice bar and line of pantry staples and adaptogen-infused "dusts" that have captivated the wellness world, Amanda Chantal Bacon worked under chefs like Suzanne Goin and as a food and wine editor at the *Los Angeles Times Magazine*, and traveled extensively across Asia and Europe studying with teachers to learn about the foods, flavors, and plant-medicine traditions of global cultures. "There is a vast, beautiful world of live medicinal foods to explore," she says, giving us a taste of it in this recipe. Amanda enjoys this hot cocoa–like drink to help relieve stress, balance energy, and give her libido a healthy boost from ingredients like *ho shou wu* and schisandra berries, which can be found online and at many natural food stores.

WELL + GOOD

HOT SEX MILK

Serves 1

1½ cups pumpkin seed milk or other nondairy milk

1 tablespoon maca powder

1 tablespoon raw cacao powder

1 teaspoon ho shou wu (optional)

1 teaspoon ghee or coconut oil

¼ teaspoon ground schisandra berries (optional)

⅛ teaspoon cayenne pepper

1 teaspoon bee pollen, for garnish

1. Warm the pumpkin seed milk in a small saucepan over low heat for 3 to 4 minutes. Carefully transfer the milk to a high-speed blender. Add the maca, cacao, ho shou wu (if using), ghee, schisandra berries (if using), and cayenne. Blend until warm and frothy.

2. Pour the drink into a mug, garnish with bee pollen, and serve warm.

DAIRY-FREE

GLUTEN-FREE

LOW-INFLAMMATION

VEGETARIAN

BETTER SEX

CONTRIBUTORS

MARCUS ANTEBI is the founder of Juice Press, an organic grab-and-go healthy food destination which has an expansive USDA organic product line, as well as a sense of humor.

DAVE ASPREY is the founder and CEO of Bulletproof 360, Inc., a food, beverage, and content company, the creator of the widely popular Bulletproof Coffee, and a two-time best-selling science author.

JESSICA ASSAF is a Harvard Business School graduate, a clean-beauty activist, and the founder of Cannabis Feminist, a female-led cannabis community, and cofounder of a hemp-based wellness company.

KSENIA AVDULOVA is the founder of @breakfastcriminals, an award-nominated digital platform merging food and mindfulness around her favorite meal of the day.

ANDREA BEMIS is an organic farmer, home cook, food blogger, and the author of *Dishing up the Dirt*.

GABRIELLE BERNSTEIN, a Well+Good Council member, is a leading voice of modern spirituality, a motivational speaker who's been a guest on Oprah's SuperSoul sessions, and a seven-time book author, including *Judgment Detox* and *May Cause Miracles*, a *New York Times* bestseller.

ROBIN BERZIN, MD, is a Well+Good Council member and the founder and CEO of Parsley Health, a disruptive primary-care medical practice in several cities, with a data-driven, whole-body approach.

JESSA BLADES is a celebrity makeup artist, herbalist, and wellness expert. She's a pioneer in the natural beauty movement with her workshops and masterclass trainings focused on wellness, cannabis, natural beauty, Ayurveda, and food-as-medicine.

JILL BLAKEWAY, LAC, DACM, is the acupuncturist-founder of Yinova, a renowned health center in New York City. The Well+Good Council member is an author and a fertility and sexual health expert.

TATIANA BONCOMPAGNI is a health and wellness writer, group fitness instructor, and mom of three based in Manhattan.

LO BOSWORTH is the actress-entrepreneur behind TheLoDown, a media brand with a focus on wellness, food, beauty, and mental health, and Love Wellness, a doctor-recommended line of women's wellness products.

BOBBI BROWN is a beauty industry titan, world-renowned makeup artist, and serial entrepreneur most recently launching Evolution_18, a line of lifestyle-inspired wellness products.

ALEXIA BRUE is the cofounder of Well+Good. She oversees the company's business functions and is a trained journalist, the author of *Cathedrals of the Flesh*, and a wellness industry expert.

NIKISHA BRUNSON is a health and wellness social media influencer and the founder of the all-natural, small-batch skincare and haircare line Folie Apothecary.

MARCO CANORA is a New York City–based chef and restaurateur, a television personality, the owner of the Hearth Restaurant and Terroir wine bar, and the founder of Brodo bone broth counters and products.

JENNY CARR is a speaker, MOM-prenuer, leading inflammation expert, and author of the international best-selling *Peace of Cake: The Secret to an Anti-Inflammatory Diet* as well as the upcoming book *The Clean Eating Kid*.

ALISON CAYNE is the founder of Haven's Kitchen, a cooking school, cafe, and event space in New York City, and the author of *The Haven's Kitchen Cooking School: Recipes and Inspiration to Build a Lifetime of Confidence in the Kitchen*.

AMANDA CHANTAL BACON is the founder of Moon Juice, a Los Angeles mecca for smoothies, adaptogenic beauty, and well-being, with a chef's commitment to superior ingredients and taste, and an herbalist's perspective on healing.

AMY CHAPLIN is a James Beard Award–winning cookbook author, former chef of famed Angelica Kitchen, and a consultant with such celeb clients as Natalie Portman and Liv Tyler.

DAN CHURCHILL is a cookbook author, master of exercise science, television host, and the executive chef at his own restaurant, Charley St in New York City.

JENNÉ CLAIBORNE is a chef, blogger, and author known for creating healthy and easy-to-make vegan recipes through her website, cookbook, and YouTube channel, *Sweet Potato Soul.*

MISTY COPELAND made history as the first African American female principal dancer with the American Ballet Theatre, one of the three leading classical ballet companies in the United States.

CHLOE COSCARELLI is recognized for bringing vegan cuisine to the mainstream as an award-winning chef and best-selling cookbook author of *Chloe Flavor, Chloe's Kitchen, Chloe's Vegan Desserts,* and *Chloe's Vegan Italian Kitchen.*

LILA DARVILLE is a Well+Good Council member. As a professional relationship coach and sex and intimacy expert, she also brings her body-positive, real-talk approach to stadiums full of women as the pleasure director of a show in Las Vegas called *Magic Mike Live.*

KARENA DAWN + KATRINA SCOTT are the cofounders of *Tone It Up,* a mega healthy lifestyle community, which includes workouts, nutrition advice and recipes, and more.

SIMONE DE LA RUE is a celebrity trainer and the CEO of Body by Simone, with dance cardio studios in New York City and Los Angeles. She's the author of *The 8-Week Total Body Makeover Plan* and is an *E! Revenge Body* trainer.

LILY DIAMOND is a writer, photographer, author of *Kale & Caramel: Recipes for Body, Heart, and Table,* and a proponent of wildness in the kitchen.

RACHEL DRORI is the founder and CEO of Daily Harvest, the direct-to-consumer brand blending health and innovation to provide delicious superfoods straight to your freezer.

JOHN FRASER is a Michelin-starred chef and the cofounder with James Truman of Nix, a new restaurant that believes eating vegetarian or vegan should involve more celebration than sacrifice.

AMANDA FREEMAN is a serial wellness entrepreneur and the founder of SLT (Strengthen Lengthen Tone), a boutique fitness studio with more than twenty locations, and Stretch*d, an assisted stretching studio in New York City.

LAUREL GALLUCCI is a cookbook author and the cofounder of Sweet Laurel, a whole foods baking company using organic ingredients for delicious grain-free, dairy-free, and refined-sugar-free baked goods.

MELISSE GELULA is the cofounder of Well+Good and a pretty solid home cook. Her background in journalism and psychology informs her wellness thought-leadership and the Well+Good brand.

ILENE GODOFSKY MORENO is a health coach, recipe developer, food photographer, and author of *The Colorful Kitchen* blog and cookbook.

JOEY GONZALEZ is the CEO of Barry's Bootcamp, the original cardio and strength interval workout that innovated group fitness and started a global boutique movement.

NICK GREEN is the cofounder and CEO of Thrive Market, the online curated grocery on a mission to make healthy living easy and affordable for every American family.

EDEN GRINSHPAN is the cofounder of Dez, a contemporary Middle Eastern fast-casual restaurant in New York City, and is also a TV personality, best known for hosting Cooking Channel's *Eden Eats* and Food Network's *Top Chef Canada.*

SOPHIA GUSHÉE, a Well+Good Council member, is the author of the critically acclaimed book *A to Z of D-Toxing: The Ultimate Guide to Reducing Our Toxic Exposures.*

SHELBY HARRIS, PSYD, is a clinical psychologist and behavioral sleep medicine expert with a private practice in Westchester, New York.

MELISSA HEMSLEY is a best-selling cookbook author and one half of the London-based Hemsley Sisters, whose food business Hemsley + Hemsley has pioneered modern healthy home cooking since 2010.

MCKEL HILL, MS, RDN, LDN, is a Well+Good Council member and the founder of Nutrition Stripped, a platform with a modern take on the science of nutrition and the art of healthy living through nutrient-dense plant-based recipes and online courses.

MARK HYMAN, MD, is a best-selling author, founder and medical director of the Ultra Wellness Center, director of the Cleveland Clinic Center for Functional Medicine, and the chairman of the board of the Institute for Functional Medicine.

KAYLA ITSINES is an Australian personal trainer and entrepreneur whose Instagram and online presence—including the ebook *Bikini Body Guides* and a meal-planning and fitness app called Sweat with Kayla—has rocked the fitness industry.

GURU JAGAT, a Well+Good Council member, is the founder of RA MA Institute for Applied Yogic Science and Technology, a Kundalini yoga school with locations around the globe, and the author of the best-selling *Invincible Living: The Power of Yoga, the Energy of Breath, and Other Tools for a Radiant Life.*

DANA JAMES, MS, CNS, CDN, is a triple-certified nutritionist, a cognitive behavioral therapist, and the author of *The Archetype Diet: Reclaim Your Self-Worth and Change the Shape of Your Body.*

KRISSY JONES + CHLOE KERNAGHAN founded Sky Ting Yoga, three studios and growing, which blends vinyasa and Katonah yoga for a fun, modern method, setting, and community.

ANNA KAISER is an international fitness expert who coaches such celeb clients as Shakira and Kelly Ripa. She's the dancer, choreographer, and founder behind AKT, a national dance-cardio-based fitness method, combining strength, toning, and more, in its growing number of studios.

NORMA KAMALI, a Well+Good Council member, is an entrepreneur who finds inspiration for her fashion collections in wellness, beauty, and women's empowerment. She's the creator of the Stop Objectification movement, which encourages women to celebrate their strength and their bodies, and the new lifestyle brand, NormaLife.

GABE KENNEDY is a chef, environmental advocate, director of culinary and innovation of the Little Beet, and the cofounder of Plant People, a wellness brand that creates CBD-based products and supplements.

JORDANA KIER + ALEXANDRA FRIEDMAN are the cofounders of LOLA, an ever-expanding portfolio of trusted products for women.

MARIE KONDO is a decluttering expert who popularized the KonMari Method, which combines principles of minimalism and joy. She's the best-selling author of *The Life-Changing Magic of Tidying Up,* and the founder of KonMari Media, Inc.

NICK KORBEE is the chef-owner at the restaurant Egg Shop, a New York City café inspired by the incredible versatility of the egg, and a Chefs Cycle athlete who regularly raises money for such charities as No Kid Hungry.

ALEXIS KRAUSS is the frontwoman of the pop duo Sleigh Bells and cofounder of Beauty Lies Truth, a website dedicated to educating consumers about the ingredients in personal-care products.

RENS KROES is a Dutch blogger, model, and best-selling cookbook author focused on preparing and eating unprocessed whole foods, which she calls "power food."

CANDICE KUMAI is a wellness chef, former model, five-time best-selling author, and host of the podcast *Wabi Sabi.*

LILY KUNIN is the plant-based health coach behind the website Clean Food Dirty City and the cookbook *Good Clean Food*; she's also the founder of Clean Market, a wellness boutique in New York City.

PADMA LAKSHMI is an internationally known food expert, model, actress, best-selling author, and the host and executive producer of Bravo's Emmy Award–winning *Top Chef.*

EMILY LAURENCE is Well+Good's Senior Food and Health Editor and a certified health coach.

ANNIE LAWLESS, cofounder of Suja Juice, is now the founder of Lawless Beauty, a luxury nontoxic makeup and beauty brand.

KELLY LEVEQUE is the author of *Body Love,* and a celebrity holistic health and nutrition coach who counts Jessica Alba, Molly Sims, and Emmy Rossum as clients.

MICHAEL LIM is the executive chef and co-owner of Chikarashi, a contemporary sea-to-table poke restaurant with several locations in New York City.

FRANK LIPMAN, MD, a widely recognized trailblazer and leader in functional and integrative medicine, is a best-selling author and the cofounder of Be Well, an expanding lifestyle, wellness, and supplements brand.

WENDY LOPEZ, MS, RD, CDE, is the cofounder of Food Heaven Made Easy, a platform for people who want to learn how to prepare plant-based meals that don't require hours of laboring in the kitchen.

MAX LUGAVERE is a filmmaker, health and science journalist, and the author of the best-selling book *Genius Foods: Become Smarter, Happier, and More Productive While Protecting Your Brain for Life.*

ELLE MACPHERSON, renowned supermodel and Well+Good Council member, is the cofounder of WelleCo, a premium wellness brand known for its plant-based organic supplements designed by nutrition experts.

ALI MAFFUCCI, the founder of the culinary brand Inspiralized, is the author of three best-selling cookbooks, *Inspiralized, Inspiralize Everything,* and *Inspiralized and Beyond.*

ELISA MARSHALL is the cofounder of Maman, a popular French-infused café and event space with multiple locations in Manhattan, Brooklyn, and Toronto.

LEA MICHELE is a singer, songwriter, best-selling author, and actress known for her role in the musical show *Glee.*

JODI MORENO, cookbook author and natural foods chef, is the creator of the acclaimed blog *What's Cooking Good Looking* and the co-owner of Neighborhood Studio, a communal kitchen, dining, and event space in Brooklyn, New York.

SEAMUS MULLEN is an award-winning chef, cookbook author, health and wellness expert, and restaurateur behind Tertulia, El Colmado, and Whirlybird + Greens.

MADELEINE MURPHY is a certified holistic health coach, shamanic energy practitioner, and cofounder and Chief Visionary Officer of Montauk Juice Factory and The End Brooklyn.

MY NGUYEN is the blogger behind *My Healthy Dish,* which features the recipes she makes for her own family as a busy mom finding ways to take shortcuts in the kitchen—without taking shortcuts on flavor.

FEDERICA NORRERI, born and raised in Italy, is a recipe developer who attended the Institute for Integrative Nutrition, the Ayurvedic Nutrition and Culinary Training, and more, to bring Ayurveda healing principles into her dishes.

DAPHNE OZ is an Emmy Award–winning television host, formerly of ABC's daily talk show *The Chew.* She is also a best-selling author, chef, and the Chief Innovation Officer at Pure Spoon, an organic, fresh baby food company.

KERRILYNN PAMER + CINDY DIPRIMA MORISSE launched CAP Beauty, the all-natural beauty site and boutique in New York City and Los Angeles. They are also the authors of *High Vibrational Beauty.*

KELSEY PATEL, a Well+Good Council member, is a Reiki expert, spiritual empowerment coach, meditation teacher, and creator and owner of Magik Vibes, a spiritual and wellness product–based company.

PRATIMA RAICHUR is an Ayurvedic physician, the owner of Pratima Spa and beauty line, and the author of *Absolute Beauty.*

DREW RAMSEY, MD, is a Well+Good Council member, as well as a Columbia University–affiliated psychiatrist and farmer specializing in exploring the connection between food and brain health. He has written several cookbooks, including *50 Shades of Kale.*

BASU RATNAM is the founder of the healthy Indian-inspired fast-casual cafe Inday in New York City.

SUMMER RAYNE OAKES, an environmental scientist, entomologist, and certified holistic nutritionist, is the author of *SugarDetoxMe* and the writer behind the plant-filled platform Homestead Brooklyn.

MIKAELA REUBEN is a culinary nutritionist and health consultant with such celeb clients as Ben Stiller, Owen Wilson, and Woody Harrelson.

MOLLY RIEGER is a registered dietitian with a master's degree in clinical nutrition who works as a consultant for several brands in the food, wellness, and beauty space.

RACHELLE ROBINETT is a holistic health practitioner and the founder of Supernatural, a New York City cafe with holistic counseling that focuses on real-world plant-based wellness.

MANDY SACHER is a pediatric nutritionist, SOS feeding consultant, author of *The Wholesome Child: A Complete Nutrition Guide and Cookbook,* and founder of Wholesome Child, a website dedicated to the improvement of overall family health and nutrition.

EMMANUELLE SAWKO is the Parisian behind the plant-based food and juice bar Wild & the Moon and the lifestyle concept store Comptoir 102.

JULIA SHERMAN is the creator of *Salad for President,* an evolving publishing project that draws a meaningful connection between food, art, and everyday obsessions.

LAURA SILVERMAN is a cook, mixologist, and founding naturalist of the Outside Institute, which connects people to the healing and transformative powers of the natural world.

LAUREN SINGER is author of the Zero Waste blog *Trash Is for Tossers* and the founder and CEO of Package Free Shop in Brooklyn.

MARK SISSON is a *New York Times* best-selling author, former world-class endurance athlete, and founder of Mark's Daily Apple, Primal Blueprint, Primal Kitchen Foods, and Primal Health Coach.

EMILY SKYE is an Australian fitness entrepreneur and founder of Emily Skye FIT (Fitness, Inspiration, Transformation), an online subscription-based service providing workouts, meal plans, and motivation.

KIMBERLY SNYDER, CN, is a Well+Good Council member and a beauty-detox expert who's written several best-selling books, including *Radical Beauty* with Deepak Chopra and the recent *Recipes for Your Perfectly Imperfect Life.* She's also the founder of Glow Bio juice bars and Solluna, a wellness lifestyle company.

LIANNA SUGARMAN is the founder and CEO of LuliTonix, which offers nutrient-dense blends full of raw, organic whole greens, herbs, fruits, nuts, and superfoods.

COURTNEY SWAN, MS, is an integrative nutritionist and traveling "real foodist" on a mission to change the way America eats.

CROSBY TAILOR is a represented fashion model, college football athlete-turned-biohacker, and the sugar-free dessert chef behind Crosby's Cookies.

LATHAM THOMAS is a best-selling author, doula, and the founder of Mama Glow, a lifestyle company offering doula immersions, education, and holistic services for expectant and new mamas.

WHITNEY TINGLE + DANIELLE DUBOISE are the co-founders of Sakara, a leading organic, plant-based meal delivery program and brand of healthy pantry staples.

TARYN TOOMEY, a Well+Good Council member, is the creator of The Class, an innovative, transformational fitness experience offered in several North American cities.

LAUREN TOYOTA is a former MTV Canada host, *Hot for Food* blogger, and cookbook author on a mission to engage an audience of young people curious about how to make vegan food fast and fun.

ALISA VITTI, HHC, AADP, a Well+Good Council member, is a functional nutritionist and founder of the FLO Living Hormone Center and Balance by FLO Living supplements. She's the best-selling author of *WomanCode* and the creator of the MyFLO period tracking and improvement app.

VENUS WILLIAMS is a mega-watt professional tennis player widely regarded as one of the game's all-time greats. She is also an author and an entrepreneur as the creator of EleVen activewear.

JILLIAN WRIGHT is a Well+Good Council member, a clinical aesthetician, the cofounder of Indie Beauty Media Group, and the producer of Indie Beauty Expo, BeautyX Summit, and Beauty Independent.

ROBYN YOUKILIS is an AADP Certified Health Coach, a best-selling author, and an expert in holistic digestive health with her coaching practice, *Your Healthiest You.*

MIA ZARLENGO, MS, RD, is a recipe developer and registered dietitian with a master's of science in dietetics and a true passion for finding ways to simplify healthy food.

TANYA ZUCKERBROT, MS, RD, is a New York City–based registered dietitian, founder of the popular F-Factor diet, and a best-selling author of *The F-Factor Diet.*

RECIPES
BY CATEGORY

	DAIRY-FREE	GLUTEN-FREE	KETOGENIC	LOW-FODMAP	
CHOCOLATE MOUSSE WITH FRESH RASPBERRIES + CACAO NIBS P. 26	+	+	+		
RASPBERRY-ALMOND MUFFINS P. 29	+	+			
APPLE + CINNAMON PANCAKES P. 30		+			
SUPERFOOD GALAXY OATMEAL P. 33	+				
HONEY-MATCHA-GLAZED DOUGHNUTS P. 34	+	+			
SAVORY ZUCCHINI + THYME CREPES P. 37	+	+			
ALMOND-BUTTER CHERRY–BERRY OVERNIGHT OATS P. 40	+				
BLUEBERRY-FIG BREAKFAST COOKIES P. 43	+	+			
SHIITAKE BACON + EGG TARTINES P. 46	+	+			
EASY HERB OMELET P. 47	+	+	+	+	
WHITE BEAN EGG BAKE P. 48	+	+			
SMASHED EDAMAME-MISO TOAST WITH SEAWEED GOMASIO P. 51	+				
NUT BUTTER + FRUIT MASH P. 52	+				
BEET TAHINI TOAST WITH AVOCADO P. 53	+				
SAVORY RED LENTIL WAFFLES P. 54	+	+			
GREEN GODDESS BREAKFAST BOWL P. 57	+	+			
BROILED GINGER-CINNAMON GRAPEFRUIT P. 58	+	+			
ROCK+ROLL GRANOLA P. 61	+	+			
ZA'ATAR-SPICED CAULIFLOWER BAGELS P. 62	+	+			
LIBIDO SMOOTHIE P. 67	+	+			
MANGO-BASIL-MINT SMOOTHIE P. 68	+	+			
TUSCAN GLOW SMOOTHIE P. 69	+	+	+		
RASPBERRY-PEACH SMOOTHIE BOWL P. 72	+	+			
PROTEIN-PACKED SMOOTHIE P. 75	+	+	+		
SIMPLY ALMOND BUTTER SMOOTHIE P. 76	+	+			
COMPETITIVE COFFEE SMOOTHIE P. 77	+	+			
STRAWBERRY CBD SMOOTHIE P. 79	+	+			
CHAI + COCONUT SMOOTHIE P. 83	+	+			
BLUE MAGIC SMOOTHIE BOWL P. 84	+	+		+	
BAHARAT-SPICED EGGPLANT WITH CHERRY TOMATOES + YOGURT P. 88		+			
BARBECUED SWEET POTATO WITH TAHINI DRIZZLE P. 91	+	+			
JALAPEÑO PANCAKES P. 92	+	+	+		
ROASTED KABOCHA SQUASH P. 96	+	+			
GAZPACHO SUPERIOR P. 97	+	+	+		
CAULIFLOWER-PARMESAN BITES P. 100		+			

LOW-INFLAMMATION	PALEO	VEGAN	VEGETARIAN	BETTER DIGESTION	BETTER ENERGY	BETTER FOCUS	BETTER MOOD	BETTER SEX	BETTER SKIN	BETTER SLEEP
+		+	+		+				+	
+	+		+						+	
			+						+	
+			+			+				
+			+			+				
+	+		+						+	
+			+	+						+
+	+		+			+				
+	+		+				+			
+	+		+			+				
+			+						+	
+		+	+						+	
+			+		+					
+		+	+			+				
+			+			+				
		+	+	+				+		
	+	+	+					+	+	
			+	+	+					
+	+		+			+				
	+	+	+						+	
+	+		+					+		
+	+	+	+		+				+	
+	+	+	+				+		+	
+		+	+			+	+			
		+	+						+	
		+	+			+				
+	+	+	+				+		+	
		+	+			+				
+		+	+	+					+	
+	+		+				+			+
+	+	+	+	+	+		+			
+	+	+	+	+		+				
+	+		+					+	+	
+		+	+		+				+	
			+			+				

	DAIRY-FREE	GLUTEN-FREE	KETOGENIC	LOW-FODMAP
SPICY WATERMELON SALAD P. 103	+	+		
SUMAC PITA, TOMATO + PEACH PANZANELLA P. 104	+			
JICAMA SLAW P. 107	+	+		
GREEN HERB VELOUTÉ P. 108		+		
CHICKPEA SALAD SANDWICH P. 111	+			
QUINOA VEGGIE BOWL P. 114	+			
HERBAL CHICKEN SOUP P. 117	+	+	+	
COCONUT-LIME BLACK BEAN STEW P. 118	+	+		
KALE SALAD WITH CHICKPEA CROUTONS P. 121	+	+		
AMARANTH "POLENTA" WITH TUSCAN KALE P. 122		+		
NUT + SEED BREAD P. 125	+	+		
TOFU-PEA DUMPLINGS P. 126	+			
COLD CUCUMBER-CHILI NOODLES P. 129	+	+		
TOM KHA SOUP WITH SHRIMP P. 130	+	+	+	
ZUCCHINI-LAMB BURGERS WITH CELERY SLAW P. 135	+			
SPICY SALMON POKE P. 136		+		
SHAVED RADICCHIO, PARMESAN + TRUFFLE PIZZA P. 140		+		
CASHEW-RICOTTA TURKEY LASAGNA P. 143	+	+		
SWEET POTATO GNOCCHI P. 144	+	+		
PULLED MUSHROOM TACOS WITH AVOCADO-LIME TAHINI P. 147	+	+		
SAUTÉED FLOUNDER WITH KALE P. 148	+	+	+	
SPIRALIZED ZUCCHINI PASTA WITH ITALIAN SPICES + TUNA P. 151	+	+		
PHUNKY CHICKEN SALAD WITH MATCHA CASHEWS P. 152		+		
WARMED LENTILS WITH POACHED EGG P. 155		+	+	
VEGETARIAN PHO P. 156	+	+		
VEGAN PUMPKIN MAC + CHEESE P. 159	+			
WHITEFISH NIÇOISE SALAD P. 160	+	+		
CHICKEN WITH CHOCOLATE MOLE P. 165	+	+	+	
GRASS-FED PICADILLO P. 166	+	+	+	
FEEL-GOOD CAULIFLOWER STEAKS WITH BETA-CAROTENE PUREE P. 169	+	+		
JALAPEÑO VEGAN BURRITO P. 170	+			
CREAMY CASHEW–BLACK BEAN ENCHILADAS P. 173	+	+		
TURKEY-LETTUCE SLIDERS P. 176	+	+	+	
GO-WITH-YOUR-GUT BÁNH MÌ P. 177	+	+		
CHIA + FLAX CHICKEN TENDERS P. 180		+		

LOW-INFLAMMATION	PALEO	VEGAN	VEGETARIAN	BETTER DIGESTION	BETTER ENERGY	BETTER FOCUS	BETTER MOOD	BETTER SEX	BETTER SKIN	BETTER SLEEP
+	+	+	+						+	
+	+		+			+				
	+	+	+		+				+	
+		+	+				+		+	
+		+	+				+			+
+			+	+	+				+	
+				+		+				
+		+	+	+		+				
+						+			+	
			+						+	+
		+	+	+		+			+	
		+	+			+				
		+	+						+	+
+	+					+				
+	+								+	
+				+	+	+				
			+	+		+				
						+				+
+	+		+	+	+					
+		+	+					+	+	
+	+				+	+			+	
+						+			+	
+	+					+			+	
+	+		+			+	+			
+		+	+	+						
		+	+	+					+	
+					+	+				
+	+			+						
	+				+	+				
+		+	+	+			+		+	
		+	+		+	+				
		+	+			+				
+	+								+	+
			+		+	+				+
+					+					

RECIPES BY CATEGORY

	DAIRY-FREE	GLUTEN-FREE	KETOGENIC	LOW-FODMAP
10-INGREDIENT RESET SALAD P. 183	+	+		
TEMPEH TIKKA MASALA P. 184				
CHOCOLATE ICE CREAM P. 188		+		
MINI GOLDEN MILK CREAM CUPS P. 191	+			
SUGAR-FREE TAHINI FUDGE P. 192		+	+	
PMS-BUSTING BROWNIES P. 195	+	+		
MINT CHOCOLATE SUPERFOOD SQUARES P. 196		+	+	
CARROT CUPCAKES P. 199		+		
PEANUT BUTTER CUPS P. 200	+	+		
KETO BIRTHDAY CAKE P. 203	+	+	+	
PICK-YOUR-FAVORITE KOMBUCHA GUMMIES P. 204		+	+	
PEANUT BUTTER–BANANA BALLS P. 207	+			
MEDJOOL DATE SQUARES P. 211	+			
CHICKPEA BLONDIES P. 212	+	+		
COFFEE CASHEW BARS P. 213	+	+		
SPICED NUT MIX P. 214	+	+		
CREAMY SWEET ONION DIP P. 218	+	+	+	
ZUCCHINI SEEDED CRACKERS P. 219	+	+	+	+
TURMERIC-TAHINI YOGURT DIP WITH ENDIVE P. 220	+	+		
COCONUT-TURMERIC POPCORN P. 223	+	+		+
ORANGE ZINGER JUICE P. 226	+	+		
LOVE POTION ELIXIR P. 228	+	+		
GINGER BEER P. 229	+	+		
GREEN BEAUTY WATER P. 232	+	+	+	+
HEARTBEET COCKTAIL P. 233	+	+		
ELDERBERRY-ROSEMARY SPRITZER P. 234	+	+		
DIY BLOODY MARY BAR P. 237	+	+		
COCONUT RUM COLADA P. 238	+	+		
ACTIVATED CHARCOAL LATTE P. 242	+	+		
BULLETPROOF MATCHA LATTE P. 243	+	+	+	
AMAZAKE P. 246	+	+		+
SWEET DREAMS SHAKE P. 249				
WAKE-UP MASALA CHAI P. 250	+	+		
BOOSTED CBD COFFEE P. 253		+	+	+
HOT SEX MILK P. 254	+	+		

LOW-INFLAMMATION	PALEO	VEGAN	VEGETARIAN	BETTER DIGESTION	BETTER ENERGY	BETTER FOCUS	BETTER MOOD	BETTER SEX	BETTER SKIN	BETTER SLEEP
+	+	+	+	+					+	
		+	+			+				
			+		+					
+		+	+			+			+	
+	+		+	+	+	+				
+			+				+	+		
+			+		+					
			+	+	+					
			+		+					
+			+				+			
+				+						
+			+			+		+		
		+	+			+				
		+	+				+			+
		+	+	+		+				
		+	+		+	+				
		+	+		+	+				
+	+	+	+	+	+				+	
+		+	+				+		+	
+		+	+						+	
+		+	+	+					+	
			+					+		+
		+	+	+						
+	+	+	+			+			+	
		+	+	+						
+			+		+	+				
		+	+							
+		+	+	+					+	
+	+				+	+				
+		+	+	+						+
			+			+			+	+
+			+	+		+			+	
+	+					+	+			
+			+					+		

ACKNOWLEDGMENTS

COOKBOOK TEAM

We first and foremost thank all of the contributors to this book. You are the people who inspire what we do at Well+Good. You are leading the wellness revolution, which starts in the kitchen!

To the entire amazing Well+Good team, you are the brightest, most mission-driven people in media. We love talking kale with you every day, testing new food launches together in the office kitchen, and making wellness the norm for people everywhere.

Allie Misch, you have mad skills—culinary, editorial, expert wrangling, recipe testing, and so, so much more. Your love and magic are all over this book. I hope you're as proud of it as we are.

Johnny Miller, photographer, fine artist, friend, joining with you to bring this book to life was a creative dream. Thank you for embracing our wellness vibe and asking among the myriad technical, light, and composition questions you considered for every photo: "Does this shot need a crystal?" We love you for it.

Rebecca Jurkevich, your vision for the recipes in this book blew our minds. Ditto your deep care in the kitchen where you wizarded the chia seeds and matcha powder into gorgeousness. Huge gratitude to witty, wonderful you and your team: Cybelle Tondu, Fatima Khawaja, and Simone Steinicke.

Rebecca Bartoshesky, you so got it. Your styling skills, your sensibility, are so Well+Good. You can set our table any day. Bring Elaine Winter.

Thank you, Justin Conly, for hustling with us every day on the shoot, often from the top of a ladder.

Props to you Rob Magnotta for bringing us a creative dream team who could see the art of these recipes.

Huge thank you to our overqualified cookbook models— Nitika Chopra, Jackson Cook, Caroline Schiff, Nicole Spencer, and Mélissa Ketchandji. That salmon wasn't going to cut itself.

To our recipe testers—Casey Elsass, Allison Malec Renzulli, Romilly Newman—thank you for many things, including helping extract our experts' go-to favorite meals from their memory banks into an actual recipe.

Amanda Englander, thank you. You prophetically saw a Well+Good cookbook wayyyy back when, and checked in every few years until we were ready to turn up the heat. Now we're cooking!

Marysarah Quinn and Mia Johnson, we so appreciated collaborating with you. You beautifully translated the Well+Good digital design sensibility for the printed page.

Thank you to the Clarkson Potter team: Gabbie Van Tassel, Mark McCauslin, Heather Williamson, Elora Sullivan, Carly Gorga, and Jana Branson.

WELL+GOOD TEAM

Special shout out to Well+Good designers Ems McCarthy, Danielle Vogl, and Jenna Gibson, who looked at every font and photo in the book; senior food editor Emily Laurence, who infused the book with Well+Good nutrition intel; Erin Hanafy, who top edited everything with us and added *je ne sais quoi* to our headnotes; and Hannah Weintraub, whose social media skills and great photo eye helped this book come to life across the intrawebs.

To Jess Muse, because we love you. You are an absolutely key ingredient in the Well+Good recipe.

A big thank you to Amy Chaplin and Laura Palese, who essentially became this cookbook's spiritual guide.

Huge love to the Well+Good Council, our handpicked health squad of wellness thought-leaders, who helps keep wellness factual, front-lines, and, of course, fun.

And all the health experts—from RDs and MDs to acupuncturists and fitness leaders—we've worked with on thousands of articles. You've championed the journalistic wellness mission of Well+Good to define and demystify wellness for a growing global community—and introduced us to a lot of great food.

To the amazing Well+Good community, made up of readers, social followers, video-viewers, attendees of Well+Good TALKS, and Well+Good Retreats, we are so grateful to you for inspiring the work we do at Well+Good.

Nancy Green and Tess Roering, whose early belief in Well+Good made a world of difference.

Linda Honan, our creative muse in so many regards. You're a true visionary, Linda, and we're honored to count you as a dear friend. And to Erika Serow, without whom we wouldn't have had the insight that this should be our first book.

Sean Moriarty, cookbook collector extraordinaire, thank you for your incredible leadership and mentorship. You ask big questions and inspire us to do big things. And Jantoon Reigersman, Brian Pike, Jill Angel, and all of our California colleagues, we love being part of the passion-driven Leaf Group family.

Melisse sends gratitude to her parents, Mark Gelula and Patricia Bloom, for all those health-food store visits in early childhood (even if I really wanted peanut butter from a jar and not a grinder back then) while also fostering a love for really great food. Your collection of cookbooks and actual use of them on busy weeknights expanded our family's culinary repertoire and gave me cooking-confidence: "If you can read, you can cook," you assured me, and I just believed.

Alexia wants to thank her parents, Nord and Suzanne, who always made family dinner a priority. They instilled in me an early love of ingredient-led cooking and culinary adventure. And I hope to pass the same along to my children, Ben and Thea, who inspire me in this work to make the type of recipes featured in this book to be the norm and simply how everyone eats, and to not be considered "healthy."

Last but not least, we want to thank our spouses because they love us and haven't minded that we've been unable to talk about anything but Well+Good since 2009. We owe you dinner.

INDEX

Copyright © 2019 by Well+Good
Photographs copyright © 2019 by Johnny Miller

All rights reserved.
Published in the United States by
Clarkson Potter/Publishers, an imprint of
the Crown Publishing Group, a division of
Penguin Random House LLC, New York.
crownpublishing.com
clarksonpotter.com

CLARKSON POTTER is a trademark and POTTER
with colophon is a registered trademark of Penguin
Random House LLC.

Library of Congress Cataloging-in-Publication Data
Names: Brue, Alexia. | Gelula, Melisse.
Title: Well+Good: 100 healthy recipes +
    expert advice for better living / Alexia Brue
    and Melisse Gelula.
Description: First edition. | New York : Clarkson
    Potter/Publishers [2019] | Includes index.

Identifiers: LCCN 2018048960 (print) | LCCN
    2018049529 (ebook) | ISBN 9781984823205
    (ebook) | ISBN 9781984823199 (hardcover)
Subjects: LCSH: Cooking. | Nutrition. | Diet. |
    Well + good. | LCGFT: Community cookbooks.
Classification: LCC TX714 (ebook) | LCC TX714
    .E229 2019 (print) | DDC 641.3/02—dc23
LC record available at https://lccn.loc.
    gov/2018048960

ISBN 978-1-9848-2319-9
Ebook ISBN 978-1-9848-2320-5

Printed in the United States of America

Book and cover design by Mia Johnson
Cover photography by Johnny Miller

10 9 8 7 6 5 4 3 2 1

First Edition